Study Guide

for

Introduction to Critical Care Nursing

THIRD EDITION

Dawn Ellen Zimmerman, BSN, RN
Graduate Student
University of Central Florida School of Nursing
Orlando, Florida

Mary Lou Sole, PhD, RN, FAAN
Professor, School of Nursing
University of Central Florida
Orlando, Florida

W.B. SAUNDERS COMPANY
A Harcourt Health Sciences Company
St. Louis London New York Philadelphia St. Louis Sydney Toronto

W.B. SAUNDERS COMPANY
A Harcourt Health Sciences Company
The Curtis Center
Independence Square West
Philadelphia, Pennsylvania 19106-3399

NOTICE:
Pharmacology is an ever-changing field. Standard safety precautions must be followed, but as new research and clinical experience broaden our knowledge, changes in treatment and drug therapy may become necessary or appropriate. Readers are advised to check the most current product information provided by the manufacturer of each drug to be administered to verify the recommended dose, the method and duration of administration, and contraindications. It is the responsibility of the appropriately licensed health care provider, relying on experience and knowledge of the patient, to determine dosages and the best treatment for each individual patient. Neither the Publisher nor the editor assume any liability for any injury and/or damage to persons or property arising from this publication.

Study Guide for INTRODUCTION TO CRITICAL CARE NURSING   ISBN 0-7216-8691-5
Third Edition

Printed in United States of America

Last digit is the print number: 9 8 7 6 5 4 3 2 1

Contributors

Christopher Blackwell, BSN, RN
Florida Hospital
Orlando, Florida
Graduate Student
University of Central Florida School of Nursing
(Crossword Puzzles)

Susan Pelliccio, MSN, RN
Instructor
University of Central Florida School of Nursing
Orlando, Florida
(Chapters 8 and 12)

Dedication

To Rob, who is my life support system.
To Jessica and Adrienne, who keep me in touch with joy, uncertainty, and hope.
To Mary Lou Sole, for the opportunity and guidance.
To the UCF School of Nursing, for opening its doors—and many others—for me.

I also want to thank Eric Ham and Barbara Cullen at Harcourt Health Sciences for their expert advice and input, and especially for their "eagle eyes."

—D.E.Z.

Introduction

Patient acuity is on the rise in all health care settings, not only in the ICU environment. Consequently, all nurses need an understanding of the basic principles of critical care nursing. The purpose of this Study Guide is to aid you, the student, in mastering the content of an introductory level critical care nursing course. As avid users of study guides, we have incorporated our favorite types of review and reinforcement exercises, hopefully satisfying a variety of learning styles. The Study Guide can also be used as a convenient review guide and a quick reference for basic critical care nursing content.

Key Features of the Study Guide

- **Learning Outcomes** reflect the objectives of the text, reinforcing your goals as a student for each chapter.

- The **Terminology** section provides a list of words and terms specific to the topic covered in the chapter. Familiarity with these terms is necessary for a thorough understanding of the review that follows.

- The **Key Points** provide an initial overview of the basic principles and normal physiology of the system covered in the chapter. In addition, this section parallels the text's exploration of the topic or pathophysiology of the specific system. Nursing assessment, diagnoses, and interventions are presented, as well as anticipated medical management of the various conditions studied.

- The **Review Questions** include an appropriate selection of True/False, Multiple Choice, and Matching exercises designed to reinforce your understanding of each chapter's content.

- **Personalize It!!** is a unique section that provides prompts for introspection and suggestions for integrating holism and "high touch" into the "high tech" arena of critical care nursing. We hope this section will reinforce your understanding of the impact of the psychological and psychosocial aspects of critical illness on the patient and family. The section also offers strategies you can initiate, even in the critical care setting, for patient and family education on measures to prevent unnecessary readmissions.

- A **Crossword Puzzle** is included in each of Chapters 4 through 17 as a fun approach to assessment of your mastery of chapter content.

- The final exercise in all chapters (except Chapters 2 and 4) is a **Concept Map**, which offers an opportunity to perform an in-depth application of the nursing process in a scenario appropriate for each chapter's focus. Anticipated medical management modalities are generally integrated in the map. This format can be further employed in the clinical setting as a framework for case studies.

- An **Answer Key** is located in the back of the Study Guide to provide immediate reinforcement of accurate responses to the various review questions. The Concept Maps are not included, since they will be individualized and should be reviewed with an instructor.

We recommend reading the textbook chapter first, reviewing class notes and handouts, and then using the Study Guide to assess and reinforce your learning. We are excited about offering this Study Guide and would appreciate your feedback and suggestions for improving any future editions.

Dawn E. Zimmerman, RN, BSN
E-mail: *ddz27744@pegasus.cc.ucf.edu*
Mary Lou Sole, PhD, RN, FAAN
E-mail: *msole@mail.ucf.edu*

Contents

Chapter 1

OVERVIEW OF CRITICAL CARE NURSING

LEARNING OUTCOMES

- Define *critical care nursing*.
- Understand purposes and functions of the professional organizations that support critical care practice.
- Describe standards of care and performance for critical care nursing.
- Identify current trends in critical care nursing.

TERMINOLOGY

- AACN
- ACNP
- ANCC
- CCRN
- critical care nursing

- critical pathways
- evidence-based practice
- SCCM
- telemedicine

KEY POINTS

❖ Critical care nursing deals with patient and family responses to life-threatening health problems, both physiological and psychological, in a holistic manner.

❖ New settings for critical care nursing include emergency departments, PACU, progressive care units, long-term acute care, and home settings.

❖ The American Association of Critical Care Nurses (AACN) sets standards for nurse competency, patient advocacy and care, and professional practice based on mission, vision, and values described in its position statement.

❖ Certification standards are set by AACN and American Nurses Credentialing Center (ANCC) and are based on the synergy model of practice.

❖ The Society of Critical Care Medicine (SCCM) is a multidisciplinary scientific and educational organization that promotes collaborative teamwork for delivery of high-quality, cost-effective acute health care.

1

❖ Issues faced by critical care nurses in the twenty-first century include:

- increased patient acuity
- growing numbers of older adults with complex multisystem dysfunction
- complex ethical dilemmas
- the importance of balancing "high touch" and "high tech"

❖ Trends emerging in the twenty-first century include:

- focus on cost containment
- evidence-based practice
- collaborative interdisciplinary relationships
- mandated outcomes
- telemedicine

REVIEW QUESTIONS

True/False

1. T   F   Critical care nursing is focused only on the patient and curing his or her illness.

Multiple Choice

1. Which of the following statements about critical care nursing is true?

   a.   Collaborative practice interferes with effective patient care.
   b.   *Critical care nursing* is defined as care rendered in an emergency department.
   c.   Technological advances have had little effect on ethical dilemmas.
   d.   Critical care nurses coordinate care for critically ill patients in a variety of settings.

2. The critical care nurse acts as an advocate for the patient by:

   a.   interceding for a patient who cannot speak for himself or herself.
   b.   intervening when the best interest of the patient is in question.
   c.   providing education to both patient and surrogate.
   d.   all of the above.

3. Which of the following is *not* a standard of professional practice?

   a.   The nurse caring for acutely and critically ill patients interacts with and contributes to the professional development of peers and other health care providers as a superior.
   b.   The nurse systematically evaluates the quality and effectiveness of nursing practice.
   c.   The nurse collaborates with the team—patient, family, and other health care providers—to provide care in a healing, humane, and caring environment.
   d.   The nurse's decisions and actions are determined in an ethical manner.

4. Advanced certification, such as CCNS or ACNP, requires both a master's degree and clinical practice in the field of critical care nursing.

   a.   True
   b.   False
   c.   Differs from state to state

PERSONALIZE IT!!

❖ In what setting do you visualize yourself as a critical care nurse?

❖ Do you believe involvement in your professional organization is an essential component of your career growth? Why or why not?

Chapter 2

INDIVIDUAL AND FAMILY RESPONSE TO THE CRITICAL CARE EXPERIENCE

LEARNING OUTCOMES

- List stressors common to the patient, family, and nurse in the ICU setting.
- Define the causes and treatment of ICU syndrome.
- Relate the symptoms of powerlessness and anger in the critically ill population to selected nursing interventions.
- Discuss the influence of individual personal characteristics on patients' responses to critical care.
- Describe the main needs of families of the critically ill.
- Discuss techniques the nurse can use to avoid burnout.

TERMINOLOGY

- anger
- burnout
- circadian rhythm
- desynchronization
- exacerbate
- ICU syndrome
- infradian rhythms

- physical stress
- powerlessness
- psychological stress
- sensory deprivation
- sensory overload
- synchronizers
- ultradian rhythms

5

KEY POINTS

❖ Critical care nurses must understand the relationship between the psychological and physiological realms of patient and family response to critical illness and the ICU environment. Risks and benefits of proposed interventions must be weighed in consideration of psychological as well as physical effects.

❖ The critical care environment has many stressors for the patient, family, and nurse; they can be divided into physical, psychological, and environmental.

- For the patient, physical stressors include pain, hunger, thirst, frightening procedures, tubes and equipment, and sleep deprivation. Psychological stressors are lack of control, dependence on others, confusion, and separation from loved ones and familiar surroundings. Environmental stressors include uncomfortable beds, 24-hour light and noise, lack of privacy, unpleasant odors, and sounds of other patients.

❖ *Desynchronization* refers to disruption of circadian rhythms; it is common in the ICU environment. An important nursing goal is to provide interventions to maintain circadian synchrony—for example, clustering activities to allow periods of uninterrupted sleep.

❖ ICU syndrome generally occurs after about 48 hours, with symptoms such as disorientation, memory loss, emotional outbursts, and hallucinations. It is brought on by sleep deprivation, sensory deprivation, and sensory overload. Patient age and history, medications, severity of illness, and electrolyte imbalances affect the severity of ICU syndrome (ICU psychosis).

❖ Interventions include reorienting patient frequently, encouraging family visits, allowing pictures and personal items at the bedside, and incorporating nonpharmacologic relaxation measures.

❖ Powerlessness is experienced by the patient in ICU, who feels a lack of control over the disease, over his or her own bodily functions and daily activities, and over procedures done to him or her. Lack of knowledge heightens the feeling of powerlessness.

❖ Anxiety and frustration result in anger, which may be directed at staff or family members. When the patient fears expressing anger, it is internalized and causes physiological consequences such as increased blood pressure and gastric acid secretion. On the other hand, anger may motivate the patient to change a damaging habit or lifestyle.

❖ For the family, serious illness can cause financial and emotional crisis. Often family members feel guilty if unable to visit frequently or support the patient emotionally. The equipment, sounds, and odors overwhelm them. Families need assurance, access to their ill loved one, comfortable seating, and updated progress reports. Reassurance that symptoms such as confusion are temporary helps alleviate family anxiety.

❖ For the nurse, physical stressors include shift rotation, mental and physical exhaustion, and missed meals. Death of patients, ethical dilemmas, conflict with physicians, lack of peer support, and constant changes in technology are just a few of the psychological stressors. Environmental stressors are chemicals, infectious disease exposure, and constant light and noise.

❖ Burnout results from all the above stressors and has four stages: (1) emotional and physical exhaustion, (2) negativism and cynicism, (3) self-isolation, and (4) terminal burnout. Stress reduction measures must be incorporated into a critical care nurse's schedule—for example, taking breaks off the unit, exercising regularly, taking vacations, and praising and supporting peers.

REVIEW QUESTIONS

True/False

1. **T   F**   In the critical care experience, psychosocial interventions are as crucial to positive outcomes as physiological interventions.

2. **T   F**   Disturbance of stages of REM and non-REM sleep will not occur if sedative/hypnotic medications are used.

3. **T   F**   Body temperature is subject to circadian peaks from 4 p.m. to 6 p.m. and troughs from 4 a.m. to 6 a.m.

4. **T   F**   Urine volume peaks from early morning to 10 a.m.

5. **T   F**   Praise by coworkers is one of the least effective defenses against nurse burnout.

Multiple Choice

1. Confusion in the ICU patient may be worsened by:

    a.   discussing other patients' conditions within hearing range.
    b.   frequently updating the patient to status and prognosis.
    c.   having a calendar and clock clearly visible.
    d.   providing frequent reorientation.

2. Which of the following statements about physical status is true?

    a.   All physical status changes relate to obvious physiological changes.
    b.   Physical status changes always develop into ICU syndrome.
    c.   Physical status changes can be related to psychological or environmental stressors.
    d.   Physical status changes relate to physical stressors of critical illness.

3. The ICU syndrome is most common in patients who have had:

    a.   a renal transplant.
    b.   cardiac surgery.
    c.   cranial surgery.
    d.   orthopedic surgery.

4. What are some of the common behaviors of a patient experiencing anger?

    a.   Avoidance of eye contact
    b.   Clenching of jaw muscles and fists
    c.   Demanding behavior
    d.   All of the above

5. Multiple studies have identified the needs of families of the critically ill. What is generally the highest priority of these families?

    a.   Financial needs
    b.   Information
    c.   Personal needs
    d.   Reassurance

6. The nurse would suspect which of the following patients to be at high risk for feelings of powerlessness?

   a. A business executive
   b. A nursing student
   c. A young mother
   d. An adolescent male

PERSONALIZE IT!!

❖ List six ways you can personally avoid burnout.

For myself:

Socially:

Professionally:

❖ What are your feelings about death and dying?

❖ How do you feel about families being present in the ICU? During a code?

CONCEPT MAP

Fill in all blank areas.

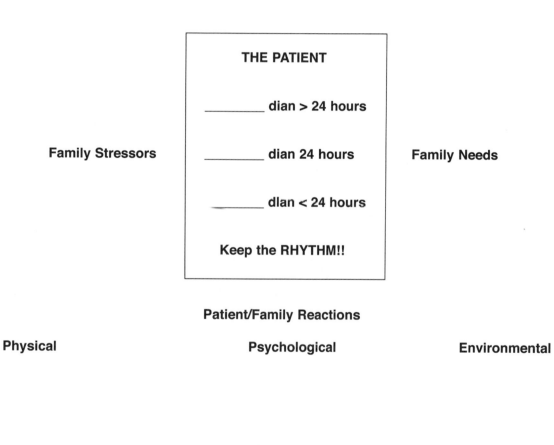

ICU STRESSORS

Physical   **Psychological**   **Environmental**

THE PATIENT

_____ dian > 24 hours

_____ dian 24 hours

_____ dian < 24 hours

Keep the RHYTHM!!

Family Stressors   **Family Needs**

Patient/Family Reactions

Physical   **Psychological**   **Environmental**

NURSING INTERVENTIONS

Physical   **Psychological**   **Environmental**

Chapter 3

ETHICAL AND LEGAL ISSUES IN CRITICAL CARE NURSING

LEARNING OUTCOMES

- Discuss nurses' ethical obligations to patients in the critical care setting.
- Compare the components of a systematic, ethical decision-making model.
- Describe the ethical and legal value of established ethical codes and standards of care.
- Define *professional negligence* and its relationship to legal professional negligence claims.
- Identify three conditions that must be present for patients to give informed consent.
- Explain how advance directives ensure patients' rights to self-determination.
- Discuss the legal and ethical issues that surround organ and tissue transplantation.

TERMINOLOGY

- abandonment
- advance directives
- beneficence
- brain death
- health care surrogate
- informed consent
- irreversible coma or persistent vegetative state
- living will
- negligence
  - acts of commission
  - acts of omission
- nonmaleficence

KEY POINTS

❖ One of the primary concerns in critical care is whether or not patients' values and beliefs about treatment can be overridden by the "technological imperative," or the strong tendency to use technology because it is available.

❖ The ANA Code for Nurses delineates the moral principles that guide professional nursing practice.

❖ An ethical dilemma involves some conflict in making a morally justifiable decision; often it centers on moral allocation of limited resources.

❖ A systematic, structured process is useful in ethical decision making. Ethical principles should always be considered.

❖ Legal accountability in nursing:

  • Negligence is the failure of a person to act in a reasonable and prudent manner.

    • Commission = a wrong action

    • Omission = failure to perform appropriate action

  • For negligence to be proven, the following elements are necessary: duty to the patient; failure to perform duty; injury to the patient; injury is direct result of failure to perform the duty. This is known as malpractice.

  • Abandonment is the severance of a professional relationship while the patient is still in need of health care.

  • In order for informed consent to be legal, competence (or capacity—ability to understand), voluntariness (consent without coercion or fraud), and information (knowledge about procedures and risks) must ALL be present.

❖ The U.S. Congress passed the Patient Self-Determination Act in 1990, requiring any health care institution that receives Medicare or Medicaid funding to inform its patients of their right to initiate advance directives and to consent to or refuse medical treatment.

❖ Durable power of attorney for health care, in which a health care surrogate is legally designated, is the most effective form of advance directive. Having some form of advance directive before a critical situation arises is the best way to avoid having treatment given or withheld against one's wishes.

❖ Extraordinary treatment measures include CPR and emergency cardiac care, as well as maintenance of life support measures, such as ventilatory assistance and maintenance of nutrition.

❖ Advanced technology has created difficult ethical dilemmas.

  • The case of *Barber v. Superior Court (1985)* brought about a ruling that both respiratory treatments and intravenous feedings are types of mechanical assistance; withdrawal of either does not constitute murder.

  • The Nancy Cruzan case (1990) was a seven-year struggle resulting in the privacy right of both competent and incompetent patients to have nutrition and hydration withheld based on a stringent test of the best interest standard.

❖ The limited supply of donated organs creates an ethical dilemma in allocation.

❖ Brain death is identified by:

  • Cessation of spontaneous breathing, spontaneous heartbeat, and all brain function.

  • These criteria are verified by:

    • No response to neurological exam and EEG.

    • Absence of cerebral blood flow in the absence of hypothermia or drug-induced states.

REVIEW QUESTIONS

True/False

1. T F   Futility is a medical situation in which important goals of care are not achievable.

2. T F   There are reliable clinical methods for determining the extent of brain damage that has occurred prior to resuscitation.

3. T F   *Barber v. Superior Court (1985)* was the basis for the ruling that respiratory treatment and IV feedings are both forms of mechanical assistance.

4. T F   There is a checklist of absolute criteria for determining brain death.

Multiple Choice

1. Which of the following statements is true?

   a. An end-stage cancer patient with extreme pain, respirations of 10 breaths per minute, and a DNR order should not be treated with large doses of morphine.
   b. A nurse who ignores a DNR order and calls a code is guilty of negligence and battery.
   c. It would be unlawful to discontinue a vasopressor drip once a patient is given a DNR order.
   d. Some institutions allow nurses to aid a physician in assisted suicide.

2. The legal term for professional misconduct that results in harm to the patient is:

   a. breach of duty.
   b. nonmaleficence.
   c. malpractice.
   d. nolo contendere.

3. Critical care nurses have a moral obligation to care for an AIDS patient when:

   a. benefits for the patient outweigh any harm the nurse might incur.
   b. the intervention is intended to do no harm.
   c. the patient is at a significant risk without care.
   d. all of the above.

4. Ideally, an ethics committee:

   a. serves to both educate and to develop guidelines.
   b. deals with generalities instead of specific issues.
   c. consists only of physicians and nurses.
   d. remains focused on protecting the hospital's interests.

5. Ordinary care generally refers to:

   a. dialysis.
   b. emergency cardiac care (resuscitation).
   c. gene therapy.
   d. care that is usual and customary for the patient's condition.

6. Withdrawal or withholding of life support includes all of the following *except*:

   a. weaning from mechanical ventilation.
   b. not starting dialysis.
   c. stopping tube feedings.
   d. stopping comfort measures.

7. Which of the following is *not* a behavior of the registered nurse as cited by the ANA Code of Ethics?

   a. Safeguards patients from incompetent, unethical, or illegal care practices
   b. Provides services with respect to human dignity and according to social and economic status
   c. Participates in efforts to maintain employment conditions conducive to high-quality nursing care
   d. Assumes responsibility and accountability for actions

Matching—Ethical Principles

1. _____ Principle of Respect for Persons

2. _____ Principle of Autonomy

3. _____ Principle of Beneficence

4. _____ Principle of Nonmaleficence

5. _____ Principle of Justice

6. _____ Principle of Veracity

7. _____ Principle of Fidelity

a. The explicit duty not to intentionally inflict harm on others

b. States that any person should be free to govern his or her own life to the greatest degree possible

c. Upheld if persons tell the truth in their communication with others

d. States that each person should be treated as a unique individual and as a member of the human community

e. Requires that health care resources be distributed fairly and equitably among groups of people

f. The duty to provide benefits to others when in a position to do so and to help balance harms and benefits

g. Claims that one has the moral duty to be faithful to commitments made to others

PERSONALIZE IT!!

❖ A 17-year-old boy, whose chemotherapy is no longer effective, is still undergoing blood transfusions that are extending his life of pain. During this admission, he grasps your hand and says, "I don't want this anymore." He understands he will die sooner without the transfusions. What would you do? What principles guide your actions?

❖ Should emergency care physician interns be allowed to practice endotracheal intubation on newly deceased patients? Explain your response.

CONCEPT MAP

Ethical Dilemma

It has been determined through diagnostic studies that Mr. Smith, 59, a heavy smoker who doesn't "believe in doctors," has severe triple vessel disease and needs coronary artery bypass surgery. His cardiologist is discouraging him from having surgery and makes a statement to you that "it's a waste of time and money —he'll never quit smoking." Mr. Smith is very fearful about having the surgery, but you know how poor his prognosis is without it, and you believe Mr. Smith lacks knowledge and evidence-based information to aid in decision making. What will you do?

Using the Ethical Dilemma Model from your text, complete the following plan.

ASSESS

Contextual Factors   **Physiologic Factors**   **Personal Factors**

Health Care Options

How will you institute the Plan of Action with:

Patient?

Family or Surrogate?

Health Care Team?

ACTION PHASE

EVALUATION

Chapter 4

DYSRHYTHMIA INTERPRETATION

LEARNING OUTCOMES

- Explain the relationships between mechanical and electrical events in the heart.
- Interpret the basic dysrhythmias generated from the sinoatrial node, atrioventricular node, atria, and ventricles.
- Describe appropriate interventions for common dysrhythmias.
- Explain the basic concepts of cardiac pacing.

TERMINOLOGY

- aberrant conduction
- asystole
- atrial kick
- atrioventricular (AV) block
- automaticity
- AV dissociation
- bipolar
- bradycardia
- capture
- depolarization
- diastole
- dromotropy
- dysrhythmia
- ectopic
- electrocardiography
- fibrillation
- idioventricular rhythm
- intercostal
- junctional/nodal rhythm

- milliamperes
- multifocal
- P wave
- pacemaker
- parasympathetic nervous system (PNS)
- paroxysmal
- PR interval
- QRS complex
- repolarization
- R on T
- sinus rhythm
- sympathetic nervous system (SNS)
- systole
- T wave
- tachycardia
- threshold
- transthoracic
- transvenous

KEY POINTS

❖ Basic ECG

- Electrocardiography is the process of creating a visual tracing of the electrical activity of the cardiac cells. The tracing is called the electrocardiogram (ECG).

- The cardiac cycle consists of the electrical activity caused by automaticity, (depolarization and repolarization) plus the mechanical response known as contraction (systole and diastole).

- The movement of the + Na ions into the cardiac cell begins the active electrical process known as depolarization. Depolarization = contraction and systole. Repolarization = resting and diastole.

- Resting membrane potential is the term for the cardiac cell's normal state of negative interior charge. It is the presence of this negative state that stimulates the formation of an electrical impulse, which begins depolarization.

- The heart can continue to generate an impulse even after blood supply and nervous stimulation have ceased. This is due to the heart's inherent automaticity, or capability to generate an electrical impulse.

  - For confirmation that cardiac systole is occurring, clinical signs, such as a palpable pulse and the presence of an adequate BP, are sought.

- The SA node is the dominant pacemaker of the heart.

- Atrial depolarization precedes atrial contraction; it is the time when blood drains from the atria to the ventricles. As depolarization ends, the atria contract and provide the "atrial kick," which increases the volume delivered by about 30%. This affects stroke volume and cardiac output.

- The wave of depolarization proceeds to the AV node, which delays entry of the impulse to the ventricles, thus allowing sufficient ventricular filling time. The AV node will take over at its inherently slower rate (40–60 BPM) if the SA node fails.

- Normal conduction pathway:

  - SA node (60–100 BPM) ⇒ Internodal pathway ⇒ AV node (40–60 BPM) ⇒ Bundle of His ⇒ L and R bundle branches ⇒ Fascicles ⇒ Purkinje fibers (15–40 BPM).

  - The right bundle branch has one fascicle; the larger muscle mass of the left ventricle requires two fascicles for adequate depolarization.

  - The Purkinje fibers have the automaticity to generate an intrinsic rhythm of 15–40 beats per minute.

- Stress, nicotine, and caffeine are common causes of increased automaticity.

❖ 12-Lead ECG System

- Provides 12 different views of the cardiac rhythm.

- Leads I, II, and III are the standard limb leads; they are bipolar (a positive lead on one limb and a negative lead on the other), and waveforms are upright.

- Augmented leads are aVR (right arm); aVL (left arm); aVF (feet). They are unipolar (record electrical flow in only one direction). They are small waveforms and so are augmented (enlarged) for analysis. Usually aVF is upright, aVR is downward, and aVL is equiphasic.

- The precordial leads (V_1–V_6) are particularly useful in the localization of anterior and lateral myocardial ischemia or infarction. They are placed as follows:

  - V_1—Fourth intercostal space, right sternal border
  - V_2—Fourth intercostal space, left sternal border
  - V_3—Halfway between V_2 and V_4
  - V_4—Fifth intercostal space, midclavicular line
  - V_5—Fifth intercostal space, anterior axillary line
  - V_6—Fifth intercostal space, midaxillary line

- None of the 12 leads records activity directly over the posterior of the heart.

- Clinical monitoring:

  - Most systems allow two leads to be monitored simultaneously. The most widely used leads are lead II and MCL_1 in 3-lead systems, or lead II and V_1 in 5-lead systems.

❖ Analyzing the ECG Tracing

- The small box = .04 sec.
- The large box = .20 sec.
- The P wave is indicative of atrial depolarization. Normal duration is 0.06–0.11 sec.
- The PR interval measures the time it takes for the impulse to depolarize the atria, travel to the AV node, and dwell there briefly before entering the bundle of His. Normal duration is 0.12–.20 sec.
- The QRS interval is indicative of ventricular depolarization. The normal width of the QRS is .06–.10 sec. Absence of a Q wave is not necessarily abnormal. A QRS greater than .10 sec. indicates bundle branch block (BBB) or an intraventricular conduction delay.
- A pathological Q wave is one that is seen post-MI and is larger than one-fourth the size of the R wave.
- The S wave is the first negative deflection after the R wave; it MUST go below the isoelectric line to be an S wave.
- The T wave immediately follows the QRS and represents ventricular repolarization.
- The ST segment connects the QRS to the T and should normally be flat. ST segment elevation or depression is often seen in myocardial injury.
- The QT interval measures ventricular depolarization and repolarization. The slower the HR, the longer the QT interval.
- If a temporary or permanent pacemaker is present and functioning, a vertical line called a pacer spike will be seen for each impulse generated by the pacemaker. If it was successful in causing a response (if it captured), a P wave or QRS complex will follow.

❖ Rhythmicity and Rate

- *Dromotropy* refers to the speed of conduction. A positive dromotrope speeds conduction whereas a negative dromotrope slows conduction.

- *Rhythmicity* refers to the regularity or pattern of heartbeats. P waves indicate atrial rhythmicity and R waves indicate ventricular rhythmicity.

- When checking for rhythm regularity, if the next beat is greater than one small box away from the proper location, it is considered irregular.

- Under normal conditions, the ventricles and the atria fire (depolarize) at the same rate.

- PR, QRS, and QT intervals must ALL be assessed for the complete picture.

- The rule of 1500 = counting number of boxes between each peak and then dividing this into 1500. The method is effective only with *regular* patterns.

- The rule of 10 = counting the number of P or R waves in a 6-second strip and then multiplying the number by 10. This method is approximate and is good for a quick assessment of rate or for irregular patterns.

- ❖ Basic Dysrhythmias

  - Atrial rhythms

    - SA node dysrhythmias

      - Sinus bradycardia (< 60 BPM) can be caused by increased vagal (PNS) stimulation (Valsalva's maneuver, gagging, suctioning, vomiting), drug effects, SA node ischemia, hypoxia, or increased intracranial pressure. It is often present in athletes as a normal finding.

      - Sinus tachycardia (> 100 BPM) is a normal response to SNS stimulation. Children under the age of 6 usually have sinus tachycardia. Other causes include exercise, stimulants, increased body temperature, and fluid alterations. It increases myocardial oxygen demand and leads to decreased ventricular filling time.

      - Sinus dysrhythmia refers to increased heart rate with inspiration and decreased rate with expiration; it is regularly irregular and generally insignificant.

      - In sinus arrest or sinus exit block, the loss of the normal waveforms creates a pause of varying lengths on the ECG tracing. This can be caused by CAD, medications, or increased vagal tone.

    - Dysrhythmias of the atria

      - Can be caused by stress, electrolyte imbalances, hypoxia, injury to the atria, digitalis toxicity, hypothermia, hyperthyroidism, alcohol intoxication, or pericarditis.

      - Premature atrial contractions (PACs): Ectopic beats are premature; PR interval is normal but differs; PACs are followed by a noncompensatory pause; the P wave is often found in the T wave.

      - Wandering atrial pacemaker: Three different P waveforms are seen; heart rate is NOT greater than 100; PR intervals vary; rhythm is irregular. In multifocal atrial tachycardia, all criteria are the same and the HR is greater than 100.

      - Paroxysmal atrial tachycardia (PAT): Occurs suddenly; HR is 150–250 BPM; rhythm is absolutely regular; P waves merge with T waves; QRS is normal.

      - The waveforms associated with atrial flutter are sawtoothed in shape and regular. Atrial rate is usually 250–350 BPM, but only part of the beats are conducted. A ratio of 4:1 or 3:1 is often seen.

- For atrial fibrillation, detection includes wavy baseline, no discernable P waves, irregularly irregular rhythm, normal to wide QRS, and presence of Ashman's beats.

  - Atrial fibrillation is particularly dangerous because of the production of mural thrombi as a result of blood agitation; these clots could dislodge once the patient cardioverts. GIVE ANTICOAGULANTS!!!

  - Ashman's beats are seen in A fib. They are aberrantly conducted beats seen with rate change and are not clinically significant.

- AV node (junctional) dysrhythmias

  - Because impulses are initiated in the AV node and surrounding tissues, P wave abnormalities and PR-interval changes are noted in junctional dysrhythmias. Impulses may be conducted forward, backward, or both.

    - When impulse moves forward, P waves are absent.

    - When impulse is conducted backward toward the atria and then forward, a shortened PR interval (< .12 seconds is seen); P wave is inverted.

    - When impulses move forward and backward, a retrograde P wave is seen after QRS.

  - Junctional rhythm: One of the above P wave abnormalities; heart rate is 40–60; rhythm is regular; QRS is normal.

  - Junctional tachycardia: Same criteria with heart rate greater than 60.

  - Premature junctional contractions (PJCs) are early beats initiated from the AV junction; P wave abnormalities (noted above); usually followed by non-compensatory pause.

- Ventricular dysrhythmias

  - Can be caused by myocardial ischemia, injury, and infarction; by hypokalemia, hypomagnesemia, hypoxia or acid-base imbalances.

  - Ventricular dysrhythmias have no P waves.

  - Diagnosis of premature ventricular contraction (PVC): Ectopic beat is premature; QRS is wider than .10 sec.; rhythm is irregular; premature beat is followed by compensatory pause; QRS is an opposite inflexion to ST (positive ST = negative QRS).

  - When the PVC occurs every other beat, the pattern is bigeminy; every third, trigeminy; and every fourth, quadrageminy.

  - The occurrence of more than 3 PVCs in a row is considered ventricular tachycardia (VT). HR is greater than 100 BPM; QRS wider than 0.10 sec.

  - Diagnosis of ventricular fibrillation: Fluctuating, jagged baseline with no discernible P, QRS, or T waves; always confirm this diagnosis with two leads.

    - Patients in V fib are in a state of clinical death; blood flow to vital organs has ceased.

  - Asystole is a complete absence of ALL electrical and contractile activities.

  - Idioventricular rhythms originate from the Purkinje fibers; the QRS is wider than normal. Heart rate is 15–40 BPM; QRS is wider than .12 sec.

- Atrioventricular (AV) blocks

  - AV blocks can be caused by CAD, infectious and inflammatory processes, enhanced vagal tone, or medications.

  - The higher the degree of block, the more detrimental the consequences.

  - First-degree block is just a slowing of SA to AV conduction. Diagnostic criteria: normal sinus rhythm or sinus bradycardia; PR longer than .20 sec.; PR for each beat is the same.

  - Second-degree type I (Wenckebach's) block is diagnosed by the following: PR progressively lengthens until P wave is not conducted; pauses are noted on ECG after P waves that are not conducted.

  - Second-degree Mobitz II block is an intermittent disruption of impulses reaching the ventricles. The PR remains constant and does not increasingly prolong (as type I above). It is diagnosed by the following: notation of occasional P waves not followed by QRS; consistent PR; regular P-to-P.

  - With third-degree (complete) block, the atria and ventricles contract independently of one another. Diagnostic criteria are the following: a difference in ventricular and atrial rates; P-to-P regular; R to R regular; PR varies from beat to beat and is not a true PR-interval; waveforms are in abnormal sequence; junctional escape rhythm or idioventricular rhythm may be present.

  - Treatments for dysrhythmias include medications, cardioversion, and defibrillation; these are covered in Chapter 7.

- Electrical pacemakers

  - Used to treat symptomatic bradycardia or to overdrive symptomatic tachycardia; may be temporary or permanent.

    - Temporary pacemakers may be transthoracic (external), transvenous, or epicardial.

    - Permanent pacemakers may be transvenous or epicardial.

  - Pacemakers may stimulate the atrium, ventricle, or both (dual chamber). Atrial pacing helps to preserve the atrial kick; dual-chamber pacing mimics normal contraction.

  - Terms to describe pacing include:

    - Rate: How fast the pacemaker fires.

    - Mode: Demand (as needed) or asynchronous; demand mode preferred to prevent pacing on T-wave (like R on T).

    - Electrical output: Amount of energy needed to initiate a contraction; measure in mAs. Transthoracic pacing requires higher mAs.

    - Sensitivity: Ability of pacemaker to recognize the heart's own activity.

  - Pacemaker rhythms noted by spike showing electrical stimulus.

  - Malfunctions of pacemaker include failure to pace (no spike when one should occur); failure to capture (spike and no impulse); or failure to sense (spike when not needed).

REVIEW QUESTIONS

Multiple Choice

1. All of the following are characteristics of myocardial cells *except*:

   a. automaticity.
   b. contractility.
   c. conductivity.
   d. myomaticity.

2. People have dysrhythmias because they have:

   a. defects in impulse conduction.
   b. defects in impulse formation.
   c. combinations of both.
   d. none of the above.

3. The normal cardiac conduction pathway is:

   a. AV node, SA node, bundle of His, Purkinje fibers.
   b. AV node, SA node, left bundle branch, right bundle branch.
   c. SA node, AV node, Purkinje fibers, bundle of His.
   d. SA node, AV node, bundle of His, Purkinje fibers.

4. When calculating the rate of a regular rhythm on an ECG, there are 20 small boxes between each R wave. Using the rule of 1500, what is the rate?

   a. 60
   b. 75
   c. 100
   d. 150

5. Which of the following statements about the T wave is true?

   a. A tall peaked T wave may signal hyperkalemia.
   b. The T wave extends from the Q wave to the U wave.
   c. The T wave immediately precedes the QRS complex.
   d. The T wave represents atrial depolarization.

6. Ventricular ectopy can be a result of:

   a. normal acid-base balance.
   b. hypermagnesemia.
   c. hyperoxia.
   d. hypokalemia.

7. Vagal nerve stimulation results in:

   a. increased atrial contractility.
   b. decreased AV node conduction and lower heart rate.
   c. increased oxygen consumption.
   d. all of the above.

8. Atrial kick is provided by atrial contraction at the end of diastole, supplying a 30% increase in:

    a. cardiac index.
    b. ejection fraction.
    c. left ventricular end diastolic volume.
    d. left atrial end diastolic volume.

9. A patient who has _____ is predisposed to atrial dysrythmias.

    a. alcohol withdrawal
    b. digitalis toxicity
    c. hyperthermia
    d. hypothyroidism

10. The sawtooth waveform of atrial flutter is caused by an irritable focus in the:

    a. atrial tissue.
    b. AV junction.
    c. sinus node.
    d. ventricular tissue.

11. Multifocal atrial tachycardia:

    a. is a result of right atrial dilation from increased pulmonary pressures.
    b. is the same as wandering atrial pacemaker, except faster.
    c. occurs often in patients with COPD.
    d. all of the above.

12. Which statement concerning use of antidysrhythmic medications is correct?

    a. Atrial dysrhythmias are not life-threatening but often require drug therapy.
    b. These drugs have similar mechanisms of action.
    c. The newer drugs have few side effects.
    d. Treatment of ventricular dysrhythmias does not affect mortality rates.

13. The following rhythm is:

    a. atrial fibrillation.
    b. atrial flutter.
    c. paroxysmal atrial tachycardia.
    d. ventricular tachycardia.

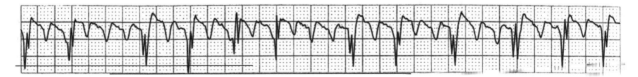

14. The following rhythm is:
    a. atrial fibrillation.
    b. atrial tachycardia.
    c. ventricular fibrillation.
    d. ventricular tachycardia.

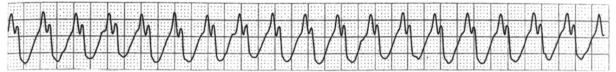

15. The following rhythm is:
    a. atrial fibrillation.
    b. atrial flutter.
    c. junctional tachycardia.
    d. junctional escape.

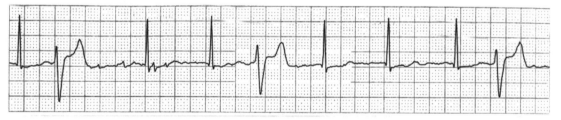

16. The following rhythm is:
    a. atrial fibrillation with unifocal PVCs.
    b. sinus rhythm with multifocal PVCs.
    c. sinus bradycardia with unifocal PVCs.
    d. wandering atrial pacemaker with trigeminy.

Fill In the Blanks

1. Fill in normal durations of the following:

    a. P wave   _____

    b. PR interval   _____

    c. QRS complex   _____

Matching—Precordial Leads

1. _____ V_1

2. _____ V_2

3. _____ V_3

4. _____ V_4

5. _____ V_5

6. _____ V_6

a. Fifth intercostal space, anterior axillary line

b. Fourth intercostal space, left sternal border

c. Fourth intercostal space, right sternal border

d. Halfway between V_2 and V_4

e. Fifth intercostal space, midaxillary line

f. Fifth intercostal line, midclavicular line

Matching—Wave Interpretation

1. _____ P wave

2. _____ Q wave

3. _____ QRS complex

4. _____ T wave

5. _____ U wave

6. _____ PR interval

7. _____ QT interval

8. _____ ST segment

a. Total time for ventricular depolarization and repolarization

b. Time for impulse to depolarize the atria, travel to AV node, then enter bundle branches

c. Atrial depolarization

d. Ventricular depolarization

e. Negative deflection immediately after P wave

f. The isoelectric baseline between QRS complex and T wave; elevated or depressed with myocardial injury

g. Ventricular repolarization

h. May represent Purkinje fiber repolarization

PERSONALIZE IT!!

❖ In your nursing education, you may not have had the opportunity to become proficient at performing a 12-lead ECG. Ask your supervisor if you can practice doing 12-leads until you feel comfortable with the procedure.

❖ Your unit's monitor technician works with rhythm strips constantly and is a great source of information on interpretation. Let your tech know you would like to see unusual rhythms and practice interpretation with his or her guidance.

CROSSWORD PUZZLE

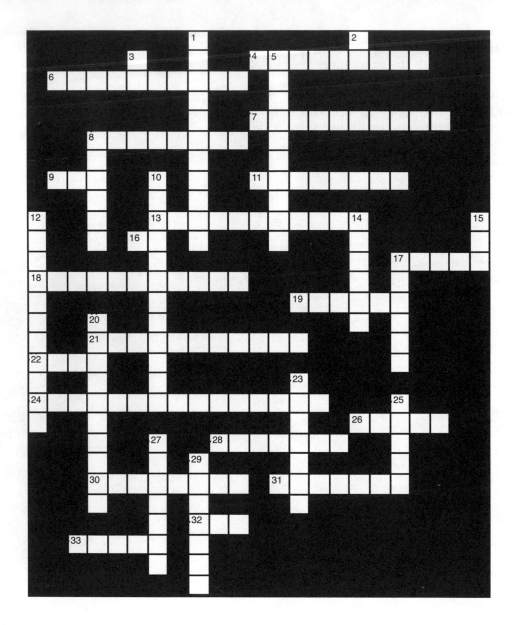

Across

4. Drug used to treat PVCs.

6. Dysrhythmias of the AV node (also known as *nodal*).

7. Second-degree heart block with progressive lengthening of PR interval.

8. PVCs that occur every other beat.

9. A quick way to calculate the heart rate is to count the number of P or R waves in a 6-second strip and multiply by this number.

11. Type of heart block that occurs when neuronal communication between the atria and ventricles is nonexistent.

13. Slowed heart rate (less than 60 beats per minute).

16. The interval is the time it takes for an impulse to depolarize the atria and travel to the AV node; normal is < .20 seconds.

17. "Normal" rhythm against which all others are compared.

18. U wave is sometimes seen in this electrolyte imbalance.

19. Type of pacemaker that "fires" only when needed.

21. Regularity or pattern of the heart beats.

22. How fast the heart is beating (normally 60–100 beats per minute).

24. Escape rhythm that is generated by the Purkinje fibers.

26. Electrical impulse of a pacemaker seen on the ECG rhythm strip.

28. Dysrhythmia with sawtooth configuration resulting from a single irritable focus in the atria.

30. Flat line on the ECG rhythm strip.

31. Three PVCs in a row.

32. Premature beat initiated in the atrium; PR interval often differs from a sinus rhythm.

33. This maneuver stimulates the tenth cranial nerve and slows the heart rate.

Down

1. Life-threatening dysrhythmia characterized by at least three PVCs in a row at a rate > 100 beats per minute; _____ tachycardia.

2. This node is the dominant, or master, pacemaker of the heart.

3. In some conditions (such as myocardial infarction, ischemia, and injury) this segment may be depressed or elevated.

5. Pathways responsible for conducting impulses throughout the right and left atria and connect the SA and AV nodes.

8. When impulse conduction through the right or left His bundle is delayed, it is called a _____ branch block.

10. Quivering of the atria with a wavy baseline and no discernible P waves is known as atrial _____.

12. Rapid heart rate (> 100 beats per minute).

14. The P wave reflects _____ depolarization.

15. Set of three distinct waveforms that are indicative of ventricular depolarization.

17. Movement of this electrolyte across the cardiac cell membrane causes depolarization.

20. Leads useful in the localization of anterior and lateral myocardial infarction.

23. Pacemaker spike followed by a QRS complex is said to have _____.

25. Degree of heart block seen as a lengthening PR interval (> .20 seconds).

27. Contraction of cardiac muscle.

29. Two PVCs in a row.

Chapter 5

HEMODYNAMIC MONITORING

LEARNING OUTCOMES

- Identify the physiological basis for hemodynamic monitoring in critically ill patients.
- Describe the indications, measurements, complications, and nursing implications associated with monitoring of central venous pressure, left atrial pressure, pulmonary artery pressure, and intraarterial pressure.
- Identify the normal values of the aforementioned pressures.
- Analyze the conditions that alter hemodynamic values.
- Explain the clinical relevance of, and the methods for, measuring cardiac output.
- Discuss the rationale and methods for continuous monitoring of mixed venous oxygen saturation.

TERMINOLOGY

- afterload
- blood pressure (BP)
- body surface area (BSA)
- cardiac cycle
- cardiac index (CI)
- cardiac output (CO)
- continuous cardiac output
- contractility
- diastole
- ejection fraction
- hemodynamics
- injectate
- intraarterial monitoring
- left atrial pressure (LAP)
- left ventricular end diastolic volume

- mixed venous oxygen saturation (SvO_2)
- phlebostatic axis
- preload
- pulmonary artery catheter
- pulmonary artery diastolic pressure (PADP)
- pulmonary artery monitoring
- pulmonary capillary wedge pressure (PCWP)
- pulmonary vascular resistance
- right atrial pressure (RAP)
- systemic vascular resistance (SVR)
- systole
- thermodilution cardiac output
- transducer

KEY POINTS

❖ Physiology

- Blood pressure (BP) = cardiac output x systemic vascular resistance (SVR).

- Cardiac output is the volume of blood that circulates throughout the body per minute.

- SVR is affected by blood viscosity, vascular tone, and endothelial friction.

- Cardiac output = heart rate x stroke volume.

❖ The Blood and Circulatory System

- Approximately 40% of the total blood volume is cellular; the remainder is plasma.

- An increase in blood cells causes an increase in blood viscosity.

- When metabolic needs increase, blood is circulated more quickly.

- In response to increased demand, the veins constrict, thus sending more blood back to the heart to enter the systemic circulation.

❖ The Cardiac Cycle

- The left ventricular end-diastolic volume is the amount of newly oxygenated blood in the left ventricle that is soon to be ejected into systemic circulation.

- This amount (above) becomes the stroke volume (SV) once ejected; that which remains is the left ventricular end-systolic volume.

- Normally, 60%–70% of the total left ventricular end-diastolic volume is ejected (ejection fraction).

❖ Cardiac Output/Stroke Volume

- Stroke volume (SV) is affected by three variables:

  - Preload is the amount of myocyte fiber stretch before the next contraction, which is controlled by the left ventricular end-diastolic volume (see also Starling Law of the Heart: more volume = greater degree of stretch).

  - Afterload is resistance to flow (SVR is common indirect measure).

  - Contractility is the force of ventricular contraction.

❖ Essential Components of Hemodynamic Monitoring

- The transducer is an instrument that turns physiological events into electrical signals.

- A heparinized solution of 3–5 ml/hr is used to keep the system patent (use of heparin depends on unit protocol).

- For accurate readings, the air-fluid interface of the stopcock is positioned at the level of the right atrium (phlebostatic axis) and the system is "zeroed."

❖ Intraarterial Monitoring

- Performed for continuous monitoring of blood pressure and ease of blood sampling for laboratory tests

- If the catheter is placed radially, perform the Allen test prior to insertion and make sure the result is positive (check ulnar pulse).

- Normal MAP is 70–100 (has to be greater than 60) and is more indicative of diastolic pressures.

- Complications of intraarterial monitoring include infection, thrombosis, embolism, and blood loss.

❖ Right Atrial Pressure (RAP) Monitoring

- Sometimes referred to as central venous pressure (CVP).

- RAP is a direct measurement of the pressure of the RA; it is indicative of right ventricular preload.

- Can be measured via central lines (e.g., triple lumen catheter) inserted into internal jugular or subclavian vein. Also a lumen in pulmonary artery catheters.

- Normal RAP is 0–8 mm Hg; a "mean" value is recorded.

- Typical RAP pressure tracing is shown as three upward deflected waves.

- Complications of RAP line placement include infection, carotid puncture, pneumothorax, hemothorax, or perforated RA or ventricle; dysrhythmias may also occur. Notify MD immediately if signs of infection occur at insertion site.

- To obtain RAP, position the patient flat and supine (or with head of bed elevated 30 degrees); read pressure at end of expiration.

- Low RAP is associated with hypovolemia, vasodilation, or any other condition that reduces venous return to the heart.

- A high RAP is associated with hypervolemia, pulmonary hypertension, or right-sided heart failure.

- Correlate values with patient assessment.

❖ Left Atrial Pressure (LAP) Monitoring

- LAP is a reflection of the LV preload and is normally 1–10 mm Hg.

- LAP catheter is not commonly used but may be inserted during cardiac surgery.

- LAP is also measured at the end of expiration.

- Low LAP is seen with hypovolemia, massive vasodilation, and high positive end expiratory pressure (PEEP).

- High LAP is seen with volume overload, vasoconstriction, and mitral valve dysfunction

- The LAP line is assessed for infection.

- A severe complication of the LAP catheter insertion is air emboli. No medications are administered through this catheter.

- Clot formation is also a complication (manually try to aspirate back into syringe).

❖ Pulmonary Artery (PA) Monitoring

- The PA catheter allows the clinician to indirectly monitor valuable information on left ventricular function.

- PA catheters have multiple lumens; catheters with four or more lumens are common.

  - Proximal lumen measures right atrial pressure.

- Proximal infusion port allows for administration of fluids.

- Distal lumen measures pulmonary artery pressure (not used for fluid administration other than flush).

- Balloon inflation port is used to inflate the balloon for pulmonary capillary wedge pressure readings (PCWP).

- Thermistor connector is used when performing intermittent cardiac output measurements.

- Newer catheters have additional capabilities of continuous cardiac output, mixed venous oxygen saturation, and transvenous pacing.

- Patient teaching is of paramount importance before PA catheter insertion.

- Catheter is inserted via subclavian (common), internal jugular (common), brachial, or external jugular vein; Trendelenburg position is used to facilitate subclavian, internal jugular, or external jugular insertion.

- Flush device system and transducers are connected to RA port and distal port for simultaneous monitoring of right atrial and PA pressures.

- Complications of insertion include hemothorax, pneumothorax, and ventricluar dysrhythmias. A chest x-ray study is done after insertion.

- The PA catheter continuously measures systolic, diastolic, and mean pressures.

  - The PA systolic pressure is the peak pressure as the right ventricle ejects its SV.

  - The PA diastolic pressure reflects the movement of blood from the PA out into the lung capillaries.

  - The PA mean pressure is the average pressure exerted on the pulmonary vasculature.

  - The normal values are 25/10 mm Hg (S/D) and 15 mm Hg (mean).

- The PCWP is measured by inflating the balloon and allowing it to float into the pulmonary capillary; it is indicative of left ventricular function.

- Normal PCWP values are 6 to 12 mm Hg.

- PCWP pressures should be measured at end expiration. Many institutions recommend reading values from a printing (strip recording) for more accurate readings.

- In patients with normal lung function, PADP is often an indirect measure of PCWP. Values can be assessed. If differences are minimal, treatment may be guided by the PADP (prevents excess inflation of balloon and may reduce complications associated with balloon inflation).

- Low PA pressures and PCWP are associated with hypovolemia.

- High PA pressures and PCWP are associated with fluid volume excess.

- Complications of PA catheters include infection, dysrhythmias, air embolism, pulmonary embolism, and pulmonary infarction.

❖ Thermodilution Cardiac Output (CO) Monitoring

- Thermodilution cardiac output is performed by connecting the thermistor to a cardiac output module or computer. A known amount of fluid (injectate) at a known temperature is injected rapidly, and the system senses temperature changes to calculate the CO. Injection of fluid must be within 4 seconds for accurate readings.

- Injectate systems are open (individual syringes) or closed-loop systems.

- Injectate may be iced or at room temperature. Current literature supports the use of room temperature.

- At least three measurements are recorded. The average of three values within 10% of one another is computed.

- Normal CO is 4-6 L/min at rest.

- Cardiac index (CI) is more valuable, because it takes body size (body surface area) into account.

- Normal CI is 2.8–4.2 L/min/m^2.

- CO/CI assists in assessment of cardiac pump failure as well as patient response to fluid administration and medications.

❖ Continuous Cardiac Output Monitoring

- Newer PA catheters have built in thermistors that allow continuous monitoring of CO/CI.

- Systems are accurate and provide ongoing assessment to guide treatment.

❖ Mixed Venous Oxygen Saturation (SvO$_2$)

- SvO$_2$ is measured continuously by fiberoptic PA catheters.

- The PA catheter measures the oxygen saturation at the distal end of the catheter.

- SvO$_2$ is a global measure of oxygen consumption and delivery; normal value is 60%–80%.

- Low SvO$_2$ results from high oxygen demands (or consumption) or reduced delivery of oxygen

- High SvO$_2$ occurs with higher oxygen delivery, when a catheter is wedged into the PA, or when tissues are unable to use the oxgyen (e.g., septic shock).

REVIEW QUESTIONS

True/False

1. T F   Cardiac output is the amount of blood pumped out of each ventricle each second.

2. T F   For accurate RAP measurements to be obtained, the air-fluid interface must be properly placed at the phlebostatic axis, located at the tenth intercostal space, midclavicular line.

3. T F   The AACN Thunder Project found heparin to be of little use in maintaining catheter patency.

4. T F   The mean arterial pressure (MAP) is a calculated pressure that closely estimates the perfusion pressure in the vena cava and its major branches.

5. T F   The major complications of arterial pressure monitoring include (1) thrombosis, (2) embolism, (3) blood loss, and (4) infection.

Multiple Choice

1. Mr. Ford is visiting the wellness clinic and has been newly diagnosed as a stage I hypertensive patient. His blood pressure assessment over the past six months has consistently been 145/92. Mr. Ford asks, "What is blood pressure?" The nurse knows that the *best* explanation of blood pressure is:

   a. "The amount of pressure exerted on the veins by the blood."
   b. "A complex measurement that should be discussed only with your physician."
   c. "A measurement that takes into consideration the amount of blood your heart is pumping and the size of the vessel diameter the heart must pump against."
   d. "A measurement that should be 120/80 mm Hg unless complications are present."

2. RAP measurements should be taken with the patient in which of the following positions?

   a. Prone, lying on the abdomen
   b. Right side-lying with the head of the bed elevated 30 degrees.
   c. Left side-lying with the head of the bed elevated 30 degrees.
   d. Supine, either flat or with the head of the bed slightly elevated.

3. Dr. Cole is preparing to insert a PA catheter into a patient's internal jugular vein. The nurse should ensure that:

   a. the patient is in the Trendelenburg position to prevent air embolism.
   b. the site has been cleaned with soap and water and is left mildly damp
   c. 50–100 mg of lidocaine has been injected prior to the procedure to prevent ventricular dysrhythmias.
   d. a tourniquet is applied to the upper arm.

4. The normal mean PA pressure is:

    a. 60%–80%.
    b. 6–12 mm Hg.
    c. 15 mm Hg.
    d. 0–8 mm Hg.

5. In order to calculate cardiac output, the nurse:

    a. takes three measurements and then calculates an average of the three if values are within 10% of one another.
    b. places the patient prone with the backrest elevated 20 degrees and records four measurements.
    c. places the patient prone with the backrest elevated 30 degrees.
    d. places the patient supine with the backrest elevated 30 to 45 degrees.

6. Mixed venous oxygen saturation reflects:

    a. the amount of oxygen perfusion taking place within the myocardium.
    b. the amount of oxygen the lungs are able to mix with the blood.
    c. the amount of oxygen attached to each hemoglobin molecule.
    d. an overall picture of the oxygen used by the various tissues and organs.

7. Which of the following complications can occur with any hemodynamic catheter?

    a. Dysrhythmias
    b. Infection
    c. Pneumothorax
    d. Pulmonary infarction

Matching—Key Terms and Concepts

1. _____ Blood pressure

2. _____ Cardiac output

3. _____ Cardiac cycle

4. _____ Preload

5. _____ Afterload

6. _____ Phlebostatic axis

7. _____ Transducer

8. _____ Right atrial pressure

9. _____ Left atrial pressure

10. _____ Pulmonary artery pressure

11. _____ Cardiac index

12. _____ Mixed venous oxygen saturation

13. _____ Intraarterial monitoring

a. Heart rate x stroke volume

b. Normal value: 1–10 mm Hg

c. Takes body size into account

d. Transforms physiological events into electrical signals

e. Invasive method for assessing BP

f. Consists of systole and diastole

g. Normal value: 60%–80%

h. Fourth intercostal space, midaxillary line

i. Normal value: 25/10 mm Hg

j. The amount of muscle fiber stretched before the next contraction

k. Normal value: 0–8 mm Hg

l. Cardiac output (flow) x peripheral (systemic) vascular resistance

m. The pressure or resistance to blood flow out of the ventricles

PERSONALIZE IT!!

❖ One of the most essential interventions the nurse can perform with a patient undergoing a PA catheter insertion is education about the procedure. The next time a patient is scheduled for insertion of a PA catheter, ask his or her nurse whether you can be present during the pre-procedural education. Watch the therapeutic communication used by the nurse and the patient's anxiety, inquiries, and overall tone.

❖ Observe the procedure for insertion of a PA catheter. Assess the waveforms and record the pressures as the catheter passes through the various chambers of the heart.

❖ Observe the nurse as she or he assesses the level of hemodynamic catheters at the phlebostatic axis and zeros/balances the line.

❖ Assess the waveforms of thermodilution cardiac output as the nurse performs these measurements.

❖ Hypertension is a prevalent illness in the United States. The next time you assess a patient's blood pressure, explain to the patient what BP consists of and illustrate the concept with the mathematical equation BP = CO x SVR. Explain the meaning of the pressure in lay terms.

CROSSWORD PUZZLE

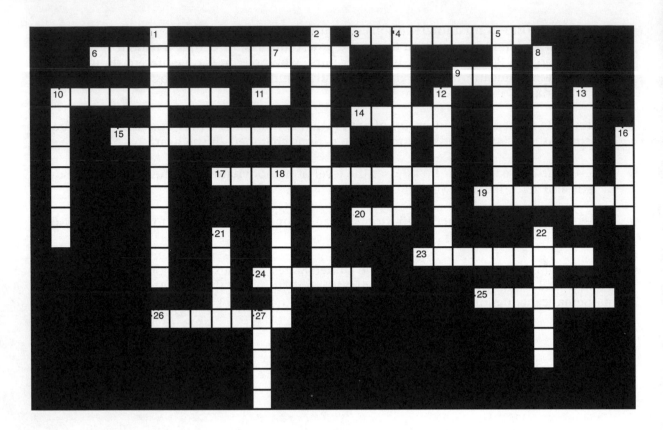

Across

3. Resistance to blood flow out of the ventricle.
6. Invasive technique used for monitoring arterial blood pressure.
9. Abbreviation for left atrial pressure
10. The _____ artery catheter indirectly measures left ventricular function.
11. Cardiac output x systemic vascular resistance (abbreviation).
14. Opening within the PA catheter.
15. Complication that occurs if the pleural space is disrupted during insertion of a central line.
17. Axis located at the fourth intercostal space, midaxillary line.
19. Flow x resistance.
20. Abbreviation for systemic vascular resistance.
23. Fluid injected into the PA catheter to measure cardiac output.
24. Tip of the PA catheter that rests in the pulmonary artery.
25. Amount of muscle stretch before contraction.
26. Surgical insertion of a central line performed because of a lack of suitable veins.

Down

1. Position of bed for subclavian and jugular PA catheter insertion.
2. Heart rate x stroke volume (2 words).
4. Part of PA catheter that measures temperature.
5. Connects to transducer via electrical cable.
7. Abbreviation for right atrial pressure.
8. Complication of arterial pressure monitoring (a blood clot).
10. Lumen of the PA catheter that is positioned in the right atrium.
12. Complication caused by violation of aseptic technique.
13. Complication of PA catheter insertion in which the balloon ruptures; air _____.
16. Measure that is calculated based on body surface area.
18. This fraction is normally 60%–70% of total end diastolic volume.
21. SVO_2 measures _____ venous oxygen saturation.
22. Part of PA catheter that is inflated to "wedge" the catheter.
27. Nickname for PCWP.

CONCEPT MAP

Following are variables that influence cardiac output. How are these variables measured, and what are normal values? What factors increase or decrease the variable?

Variables Affecting Cardiac Output	Physiologic Measure/ Normal Values	Factors That Increase	Factors That Decrease
Heart rate			
Left Ventricular Preload			
Left Ventricular Afterload			
Right Ventricular Preload			
Right Ventricular Afterload			
Contractility			

Chapter 6

VENTILATORY ASSISTANCE

LEARNING OUTCOMES

- Review the anatomy and physiology of the respiratory system.
- Describe methods for assessing the respiratory system, including physical assessment, interpretation of arterial blood gases, and noninvasive techniques.
- Compare commonly used oxygen delivery devices.
- Discuss methods for maintaining an open airway.
- Identify indications for initiation of mechanical ventilation.
- Describe types and modes of mechanical ventilation.
- Relate complications associated with mechanical ventilation.
- Explain methods for weaning patients from mechanical ventilation.
- Formulate a plan of care for the mechanically ventilated patient.

TERMINOLOGY

- arterial blood gases (ABGs)
- assist-control ventilation
- barotrauma
- compliance
- continuous blood gas monitoring
- continuous positive airway pressure (CPAP)
- diffusion
- endotracheal suction
- endotracheal tube
- end-tidal carbon dioxide monitoring
- fraction of inspired oxygen (FiO$_2$)

- functional residual capacity (FRC)
- hyperoxygenation
- in-line suction
- intubation
- mainstem bronchus
- microprocessor ventilator
- negative inspiratory force (pressure)
- noninvasive positive pressure ventilation
- oxyhemoglobin dissociation curve
- positive end expiratory pressure (PEEP)
- pressure support

- pulse oximetry
- resistance
- synchronized intermittent mandatory ventilation (SIMV)
- tension pneumothorax
- terminal weaning
- tidal volume
- tracheostomy
- ventilation
- ventilator-associated pneumonia (VAP)
- vital capacity
- weaning
- work of breathing (WOB)

KEY POINTS

❖ Review of Respiratory Anatomy and Physiology

- Oxygen and carbon dioxide are exchanged via the respiratory system to provide adequate oxygen to the cells and to remove excess carbon dioxide from the cells.

- The upper airway, lower airway, and lungs are structures involved in gas exchange.

- The process of gas exchange consists of (1) ventilation, (2) diffusion at pulmonary capillaries, (3) perfusion (transportation), and (4) diffusion to the cells.

- The rate, depth, and rhythm of respirations are controlled by respiratory centers in the medulla and pons.

- High carbon dioxide levels provide the stimulus to breathe; in patients with chronically high CO_2 levels, low oxygen levels stimulate breathing.

- The work of breathing (WOB) is the amount of effort required for the maintenance of a given level of ventilation.

- Compliance is a measure of the distensibility, or stretchability, of the lung and chest wall; it is determined by the amount of elastic recoil that must be overcome before lung inflation can occur.

- Resistance refers to the opposition to gas flow in the airways.

❖ Physical Exam

- History is important to determine etiology of respiratory symptoms.

- Physical exam includes inspection of head, neck, fingers, and chest; and observation of respirations and breathing patterns.

- Inspection provides an initial clue for potential acute and chronic respiratory problems. The head, neck, fingers, and chest are inspected for abnormalities.

- Lung sounds are auscultated routinely in the critical care setting. Vesicular breath sounds are the normal breath sounds heard over the peripheral lung fields.

- Adventitious lung sounds include crackles, wheezing, and pleural friction rubs. Crackles usually indicate fluid in the alveoli and airways. Wheezes result from rapid passage of air through narrow airways. A pleural friction rub indicates inflammation.

❖ Arterial Blood Gas (ABG) Interpretation

- ABGs monitor oxygenation (PaO_2 and SaO_2), ventilation ($PaCO_2$), and acid-base status. It is important for the nurse to assess ABGs quickly.

- Early signs of hypoxemia are neurologic, such as restlessness and anxiety.

- Cyanosis is a late sign of hypoxemia.

- Normal values:

  - PaO_2 80–100 mm Hg

  - SaO_2 93%–99%; values above 90% are often considered adequate in the critically ill patient.

  - $PaCO_2$ 35–45 mm Hg; think of as acid

- HCO_3 22–26 mEq/L; think of as acid neutralizer

- pH 7.35–7.45

- SaO_2 of 90% = PaO_2 of 60 mm Hg

- Steps in ABG Interpretation:

  - Step 1—Evaluate oxygenation

  - Step 2—Evaluate acid-base status: Look at pH, $PaCO_2$, and HCO_3

  - Step 3—Determine primary acid-base imbalance: What is the main cause of the imbalance?

  - Step 4—Determine compensation: Did the body attempt to compensate for the imbalance? Compensation can be none, partial (pH still abnormal), or complete

- Common acid-base abnormalities:

  - Respiratory acidosis—retention of carbon dioxide (hypoventilation)

  - Respiratory alkalosis—excess elimination of carbon dioxide (hyperventilation)

  - Metabolic acidosis—gain of metabolic acids or loss of base (renal failure, diabetic ketoacidosis, diarrhea)

  - Metabolic alkalosis—gain of base or loss of metabolic acids (vomiting, nasogastric suction, antacids)

❖ Noninvasive Assessment of Gas Exchange

- Pulse oximetry is commonly used in critical care setting and gives continuous value for oxygen saturation.

- End-tidal carbon dioxide monitoring is commonly used to trend values.

- Both measures are useful in reducing the number of ABGs.

❖ Oxygen Administration

- If oxygen levels are low, supplemental oxygen is given.

- Commonly used oxygen delivery devices include the nasal cannula, the facemask, the facemask with reservoir, and the Venturi mask.

- Masks with reservoirs provide the greatest concentration of oxygen.

- Venturi masks more accurately deliver smaller amounts of oxygen and are good for patients with chronic lung disease.

- A bag-valve-mask device is used in emergencies to ventilate the patient; supplemental oxygen (15 L/min) is given through the device in attempt to administer 100% oxygen.

❖ Maintaining an Open Airway

- Oral airways are rigid tubes that prevent the tongue from falling into the pharynx; they are not tolerated in an alert patient.

- Nasopharyngeal airways are softer tubes inserted through the nose. They can facilitate nasotracheal suctioning in patients with ineffective airway clearance. High risk for sinusitis exists with these airways.

❖ Endotracheal Intubation and Tracheostomies

- Intubation is the insertion of an endotracheal tube (ETT) into the trachea through either the mouth or the nose.

- ETTs used in adults have a balloon or cuff to facilitate ventilation and prevent aspiration.

- Ventilation is performed with a bag-valve device or a mechanical ventilator connected to the ETT.

- Intubation is performed by a trained individual; it should be completed within 30 seconds.

- The nurse assists in intubation by gathering equipment, suctioning the oropharynx prior to intubation, suctioning the ETT after intubation, and validating tube placement.

- Auscultating over the epigastric area and lung fields validates correct placement of ETT; an end-tidal carbon dioxide detector can also help to verify tube placement.

- A tracheostomy is done for long-term ventilatory management and/or secretion removal.

- Patients with ETT and tracheostomies require suctioning to clear the airway.

- Suctioning is done on an as-needed basis.

- Duration of suction should not exceed 15 seconds.

- Patients are hyperoxygenated prior to the procedure; this is best done via the suction mode on the ventilator.

- Closed, or in-line, suction devices are used to maintain oxygenation during the suction procedure.

- Normal saline should not be routinely instilled into the artificial airway during the suction procedure; research has shown that it increases the likelihood of oxygen desaturation associated with suctioning.

❖ Mechanical Ventilation

- Mechanical ventilation is used as a supportive therapy to facilitate gas exchange. Most methods require an artificial airway (endotracheal tube or tracheostomy). Noninvasive techniques may be used to augment gas exchange in selected populations.

- Negative pressure ventilation is used for individuals with chronic respiratory failure who require assisted ventilation for short periods; examples of negative-pressure respirators are the cuirass and poncho.

- Noninvasive positive pressure ventilation is used to manage chronic respiratory failure and acute respiratory failure that is expected to resolve quickly—e.g., pulmonary edema.

- Positive pressure ventilation (PPV) is commonly used in critically ill patients; newer ventilators incorporate microprocessors to facilitate ventilation.

- Volume targeted ventilation is a type of PPV in which the ventilator gives a preset volume of gases.

- Pressure-targeted ventilation is a type of PPV that delivers gases until a preset pressure is reached.

❖ Volume-Targeted Modes of Mechanical Ventilation

- Controlled ventilation provides ventilation regardless of patient effort; this method is rarely used.

- Assist/control ventilation delivers a preset VT whenever the patient exerts a negative inspiratory effort.

- Synchronized intermittent mandatory ventilation (SIMV) delivers a preset VT at a preset respiratory rate and permits the patient to breathe spontaneously at his or her own respiratory rate and depth between the ventilator breaths.

- Pressure support ventilation augments spontaneous breathing efforts with positive pressure.

❖ Adjuncts to Mechanical Ventilation

- Positive end expiratory pressure (PEEP) adds pressure at the end of expiration to prevent the collapse of small airways, increases functional residual capacity (FRC), and improves oxygenation.

- Common side effects of PEEP therapy are barotrauma and decreased cardiac output.

- Continuous positive airway pressure (CPAP) is used to augment FRC during spontaneous ventilation.

❖ Key Nursing Interventions for Mechanically Ventilated Patients

- Maintain airway.

- Be prepared for emergencies.

- Perform mouth care routinely; inspect the mouth and mucous membranes, especially around the ETT.

- Assist in relief of anxiety; patient may need medications.

- Neuromuscular blockade is used to chemically paralyze patients with severe respiratory failure; it may assist in tolerating the nontraditional modes of ventilation.

- Patients on neuromuscular blockers must always be sedated, and the level of blockage is assessed with the train-of-four technique using a peripheral nerve stimulator.

- Prevent accidental extubation.

- Establish means of communication with patient.

- Maintain adequate nutrition; tube feedings are commonly administered; prevent/assess for aspiration.

- The nurse should be able to assess the following settings on the ventilator: mode, tidal volume, respiratory rate, FiO_2, peak inspiratory pressure.

❖ Complications of Mechanical Ventilation

- Barotrauma is the presence of extraalveolar air. The most common barotrauma complication is pneumothorax.

- Tension pneumothorax is life-threatening; air accumulates in the pleural space and causes cardiopulmonary collapse; immediate needle thoracostomy or chest tube insertion is essential

- Monitor peak inspiratory pressures

- ETT may migrate into the right mainstem bronchus; auscultate for bilateral breath sounds routinely and after manipulation of ETT.

- Cuff pressures on the ETT and tracheostomy are monitored; excess pressures can cause tracheal damage while pressures that are too low cause air to leak around, and may promote aspiration. Pressures in the cuff should not exceed 30 cm H2O.

- Aspiration is a common complication related to tube feedings and inadequate pressure in the cuff of the artificial airway. Patients need to have the head of bed elevated for feedings. Gastric residuals should be assessed every four hours.

- All mechanically ventilated patients are at high risk for ventilator-associated pneumonia. Hand washing and meticulous care of ventilator equipment can assist in preventing pneumonia.

- High levels of PEEP are associated with a decrease in cardiac output related to decreased venous return.

- Patients can become psychologically dependent on the ventilator.

❖ Troubleshooting the Ventilator

- *Never shut off alarms.*

- Manually ventilate the patient with a bag-valve-mask device if unable to troubleshoot alarms quickly.

- Keep a bag-valve-mask device at the bedside.

- A low exhaled volume alarm sounds if the patient does not receive the preset VT (e.g., from disconnections).

- A high-pressure alarm occurs if the preset pressure limit is exceeded; this usually occurs if something is obstructing flow such as coughing, secretions, or kinked ETT or ventilator tubing.

- An apnea alarm occurs if the ventilator does not detect spontaneous respiration within a present interval.

❖ Weaning Patients From Mechanical Ventilation

- Weaning from mechanical ventilation is a challenge.

- Patients must be physically and psychologically ready to wean. Weaning indices and assessment parameters can assist in predicting readiness to wean.

- Several factors are essential prior to weaning the patient from mechanical ventilation: underlying cause must be resolved; hemodynamic stability, adequate respiratory muscle strength, and adequate nutrition must be ensured; patient must be alert and without pain; there must be no infection, anemia, or other problems that increase oxygen demand and the work of breathing.

- Psychological support is essential during the weaning process.

- Weaning is discontinued if patient exhibits signs of respiratory distress or if oxygen saturation deteriorates.

- Weaning from short-term ventilation can be done by using a T-piece or reducing the SIMV rate.

- Weaning from long-term ventilation is often difficult.

- Two approaches to weaning long-term patients:

  - High-pressure, low-volume work promotes conditioning. Strategies include T-piece trials that gradually increase the amount of time off the ventilator, low SIMV rates, and the use of CPAP trials.

  - Low-pressure, high-volume work promotes endurance. Pressure support ventilation is used.

- Terminal weaning may be done to withdraw mechanical ventilation from a terminally ill patient. Comfort measures and psychological support are essential.

REVIEW QUESTIONS

True/False

1. T F Mechanical ventilation is commonly used in critical care settings and is not associated with complications.

2. T F Respiratory acidosis occurs if the patient hyperventilates.

3. T F Pulse oximetry is used to measure arterial oxygen saturation noninvasively.

4. T F An end-tidal CO_2 detector assists in verifying endotracheal tube placement.

5. T F Ventilator-associated pneumonia can be prevented by suctioning the patient every two hours.

6. T F Saline should be routinely instilled into endotracheal tubes to loosen secretions from the respiratory tract.

Multiple Choice

1. Compliance increases with:

   a. ARDS.
   b. emphysema.
   c. obesity.
   d. pulmonary fibrosis.

2. Normal respirations are stimulated by:

   a. acidotic pH.
   b. high carbon dioxide levels.
   c. low oxygen levels.
   d. low serum bicarbonate levels.

3. A $PaCO_2$ greater than 45 mm Hg indicates:

   a. metabolic acidosis.
   b. metabolic alkalosis.
   c. respiratory acidosis.
   d. respiratory alkalosis.

4. If the low-exhaled volume alarm is sounding, the nurse should:

   a. assess to see that the ventilator is attached to the endotracheal tube.
   b. extubate the patient.
   c. see whether the patient is biting the endotracheal tube.
   d. set the tidal volume at a higher level.

5. Weaning from long-term mechanical ventilation:

   a. is easily done over several hours using a T-piece.
   b. is not affected by fever or abdominal distention.
   c. often combines T-piece trials, SIMV, and pressure support.
   d. should not be attempted if the patient's family is present in the room.

6. Assess the following arterial blood gases:

   pH—7.48, $PaCO_2$—33 mm Hg, HCO_2—20 mEq/L, PaO_2 85 mm Hg
   a. Fully compensated metabolic acidosis; normal oxygenation
   b. Normal ABGs
   c. Partly compensated respiratory acidosis with hypoxemia
   d. Uncompensated respiratory alkalosis; normal oxygenation

Matching—Key Terms

1. _____ In-line suction

2. _____ Assist/control ventilation

3. _____ PEEP

4. _____ T-piece trial

5. _____ Neuromuscular blockade

6. _____ Intubation

7. _____ Noninvasive ventilation

8. _____ Bag-valve-mask device

a. Provides short-term ventilatory support, such as treatment of acute pulmonary edema

b. Insertion of endotracheal tube

c. Closed-system; method of aspirating secretions while keeping the patient ventilated

d. Paralyzes the respiratory muscles to facilitate ventilation

e. Used to ventilate a patient manually

f. Increases functional residual capacity

g. Method of weaning from mechanical ventilation

h. Positive pressure ventilation that ensures a preset rate at a preset volume

PERSONALIZE IT!!

❖ Talk to a patient who has recently undergone mechanical ventilation and is now weaned from the ventilator. Ask the patient what he or she remembers about the experience and how nurses facilitated the procedure.

❖ Think about alternatives to physical restraints in preventing accidental extubation.

❖ Observe nurses and respiratory therapists in the critical care unit as they manage patients who require mechanical ventilation; look at the charting that is done to record and monitor the patient's status.

CROSSWORD PUZZLE

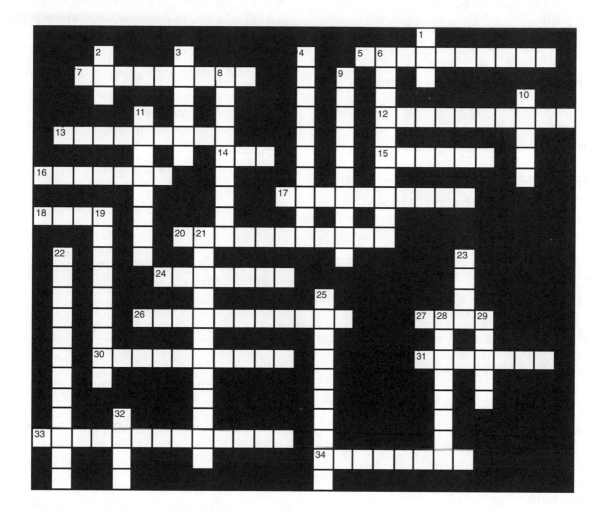

Across

5. Opposition to gas flow in the airways.
7. Sounds normally heard over the large central airways.
12. Insertion of an endotracheal tube.
13. Adult respiratory rate > 20 breaths per minute.
14. Increased intrathoracic pressure associated with PEEP may result in a ___ cardiac output.
15. _____-control ventilation is a mode that delivers preset number of breaths each minute at a preset volume.
16. Process for withdrawing patients from mechanical ventilation.
17. Procedure to remove mucus from the airways.
18. Mode for mechanical ventilation that allows the patient to take spontaneous breaths in between machine breaths (abbreviation).
20. _____ acidosis is a condition in which carbon dioxide is retained and pH falls < 7.35.
24. Besides the pons, this area of the brain also controls vital centers responsible for breathing.
26. Movement of gases into and out of the alveoli.
27. Abbreviation for a noninvasive method for providing mechanical ventilation.
30. Patients with artificial airways who receive tube feedings are at risk for this complication.
31. Mask that can deliver high flow of oxygen at a fixed concentration.
33. It is important to establish a method of _____ with the ventilated patient.
34. Formerly called *rales*.

Down

1. Abbreviation of negative inspiratory pressure.
2. Volume of gas remaining in the lungs at normal resting expiration (abbreviation).
3. _____-Stokes respirations are cyclical and become increasingly shallow until a period of apnea lasting approximately 20 seconds occurs.
4. Presence of extraalveolar air.
6. _____ reserve volume is the maximum amount of gas forcefully expired at the end of a normal breath.
8. Respiratory _____ results when carbon dioxide is hyperexcreted from the lungs and pH rises > 7.45.
9. Removal of the endotracheal tube.
10. Volume of a normal breath (normally 500 ml).
11. Late sign of hypoxemia that should not be relied upon as an early indicator of respiratory distress.
19. Breath sounds over the peripheral lung fields.
21. A(n) _____ tube is inserted into airway to facilitate ventilation.
22. Instrument used to visualize the vocal cords for insertion of an endotracheal tube.
23. Abbreviation for added pressure that prevents collapse of the alveoli at the end of expiration.
25. Measure of the "stretchability" of the lung and chest wall.
28. "Support" that helps to decrease the work of breathing.
29. _____ capacity measures the volume of gas that can be forcefully expired after maximum inspiration.
32. Part of an endotracheal tube or tracheostomy that "seals off" the airway.

CONCEPT MAP

Observe a patient who is receiving mechanical ventilation.

Respiratory Assessment   **Reasons for Mechanical Ventilation**

ABGs
pH _____
$PaCO_2$ _____
HCO_3 _____
PaO_2 _____
O_2 sat _____

Interpretation of ABGs _____

Possible causes of abnormalities _____

Anticipated intervention(s) for ABG abnormalities _____

Assessment of Readiness to Wean From Mechanical Ventilation

Positive Factors   Potential Factors That Prohibit Weaning

Plans for Weaning From Mechanical Ventilation

Physical   Psychosocial

Chapter 7

CODE MANAGEMENT

LEARNING OUTCOMES

- Compare roles of caregivers in managing cardiopulmonary arrest situations.
- Identify equipment used during a code.
- Differentiate basic and advanced life support measures used during a code.
- Identify medications used in code management, including use, action, side effects, and nursing implications.
- Discuss treatment of special problems that can occur during a code.
- Describe special concerns related to the geriatric population during a code.
- Identify information to be documented during a code.
- Describe care of patients after resuscitation.
- Identify psychosocial, legal, and ethical issues related to code management.

TERMINOLOGY

- advanced cardiac life support (ACLS)
- ACLS algorithm
- automatic implantable cardiovertor defibril-lator (AICD)
- automatic external defibrillator (AED)
- basic life support (BLS)
- cardioversion
- code/arrest
- crash cart

- defibrillation
- external pacer
- joules/watt seconds
- paradoxical pulse
- Patient Self-Determination Act (PSDA)
- pericardial tamponade
- pericardiocentesis
- tension pneumothorax

KEY POINTS

❖ The Code Team

- The person who recognizes cardiopulmonary arrest calls a code, then performs one-person CPR until help arrives.

- The person who runs or directs the code is responsible for making diagnostic and treatment decisions—usually a physician.

- The primary nurse provides information to the code director, contacts attending physician, and assists with medications and procedures.

- The second nurse coordinates use of the crash cart, prepares and labels meds, and assembles equipment for procedures.

- The nursing supervisor limits the number of people present, communicates with the family, and coordinates transfer to ICU.

- The anesthesiologist or CRNA assumes control of ventilation and oxygenation.

- The respiratory therapist assists with ventilation, performs ABGs, suctioning, and may intubate if trained.

- Some code teams include a pharmacist or pharmacy tech to assist with medication preparation and restocking of crash cart medications afterwards.

❖ Equipment Used in Codes

- Cardiac board, monitor-defibrillator

- Bag-valve device (BVD) with supplemental oxygen at 100%

- Normal saline and Ringer's lactate solutions (commonly used)

❖ Resuscitation

- Resuscitation efforts begin with BCLS (basic cardiac life support).

  - ABCs of CPR = *A*irway, *B*reathing, and *C*irculation.

  - Brain damage may occur in 4–6 minutes without adequate oxygen.

  - Improper head position is the most common cause of inability to ventilate.

- Once assistance arrives, ACLS protocol is followed.

  - ABCDs of ACLS = *A*irway, *B*reathing, *C*irculation, and *D*efibrillation.

  - The primary survey consists of the ABCs plus early defibrillation.

- At defibrillation, the secondary survey is initiated.

  - The secondary survey extends the above ABCDs by one more D: the differential diagnosis—with more in-depth assessments and interventions.

  - Intubation with an endotracheal tube (ETT) is recommended before gaining IV access. CPR should not be interrupted for longer than 30 seconds while ETT is placed.

  - ETT placement is verified first by making sure air is not heard in the epigastrum. Check for bilateral breath sounds and get an X-ray.

- Use end-tidal CO_2 or esophageal detector as a secondary method to confirm ETT placement.

- Circulation focuses on IV access, electrode and lead placement, rhythm identification, blood pressure monitoring, and administration of medications.

- Medications that can be administered via ETT before IV access are epinephrine, lidocaine, and atropine. They should be mixed in preservative-free NS (normal saline): epinephrine and lidocaine at 2–2.5 times the IV dose diluted in 10 ml NS; atropine 2–3 mg diluted in NS.

- When medications are administered peripherally by IV push, they should be followed with a 20–30 ml NS flush.

- Differential diagnosis involves the "why" of the arrest. If a reversible cause is identified, specific therapy can be initiated. Lethal dysrhythmias must be identified: V fib/V tach, asystole, and pulseless electrical activity (PEA). Symptomatic bradycardias and tachycardias are also treated.

❖ Recognition and Treatment of Dysrhythmias (while continuing CPR)

- For V fib or pulseless V tach:

  - Initiate ABCDs.

  - Defibrillate ASAP.

  - Defibrillate up to 3 times in rapid succession if needed.

  - Assess for pulse. If still no pulse, continue CPR, intubate, access IV.

  - Administer epinephrine (Epi) 1 mg IV push q 3–5 minutes; defibrillate at 360 joules (J) within 30 seconds of each Epi dose.

  - Vasopressin 40 units IV (1 dose) is an option for epinephrine.

  - Other drugs that may be used: amiodarone, lidocaine, magnesium, procainamide, or bicarb; sequence is "drug-shock."

  - Reassess patient frequently!

- For PEA:

  - Determine and treat underlying cause (hypovolemia, hypoxia, cardiac tamponade, tension pneumothorax, drug overdose (OD), pulmonary embolism, acidosis, MI, or hypothermia).

  - Administer Epi 1 mg IVP q 3–5 min.

  - May give atropine 1 mg IV q 3–5 minutes up to max 0.04 mg/kg for bradycardia.

- For asystole:

  - Determine and treat underlying cause (hypoxia, hyper- or hypokalemia, preexisting acidosis, drug overdose, or hypothermia).

  - Consider transcutaneous pacing; administer Epi 1 mg IVP q 3–5 minutes, atropine 1 mg IV q 3–5 minutes up to max 0.04 mg/kg.

- For symptomatic bradycardia:

  - Start by administering atropine 0.5–1 mg IVP.

- Consider transcutaneous pacing.

- Give dopamine for blood pressure (BP) support.

- DO NOT GIVE LIDOCAINE.

- For symptomatic tachycardias: (A fib, A flutter, SVT, wide-QRS tachycardia, and VT)

  - Adenosine may be given.

  - Synchronized cardioversion and antidysrhythmic therapy may be needed.

  - Sedate prior to cardioversion if possible.

  - Low energy levels (50 J) are often sufficient for A flutter and SVT.

❖ Electrical Therapy—Definitions

- Defibrillation: "countershock" completely depolarizes the heart so that SA node or other pacemaker can resume control; may use external paddles (hands on), electrode pads (hands off), or smaller internal paddles during cardiac surgery.

- AED (automatic external defibrillators): external defibrillators with rhythm analysis capability; can be used by BLS trained personnel and laypersons.

- Cardioversion: synchronous shock delivered during ventricular depolarization, on the R-wave; disrupts rather than completely depolarizes the rhythm; less energy required; paddles must remain depressed until shock is delivered; sedation decreases discomfort.

- Transcutaneous cardiac pacing: emergency treatment of symptomatic bradycardia and asystole; external and noninvasive; a temporary measure.

- ICD (implantable cardioverter defibrillator) or permanent pacemaker: paddles should not be placed over the generator; anterior-posterior (AP) paddle placement is better; external defibrillation does not harm the patient, ICD, or pacemaker.

❖ Special Problems Encountered During a Code

- Tension pneumothorax—symptoms of dyspnea, chest pain, tachypnea, and tachycardia; life-threatening; air enters the pleural space and cannot escape.

- Pericardial tamponade—accumulation of fluid in the pericardial sac leads to decreased cardiac output; PEA or arrest may follow.

❖ Detailed documentation is essential during a code!

❖ After the resuscitation, the patient is transferred to ICU; family must receive honest prognosis. Ideally, end-of-life preferences have been discussed with family prior to critical situation.

REVIEW QUESTIONS

True/False

1. T F A patient should always be tapped or shaken and asked, "Are you OK?" before initiating life support measures.

2. T F Improper mask position is the most common cause of inability to ventilate a patient.

3. T F On an average adult, chest compressions depress the sternum by 2 to 3 inches.

4. T F BLS providers are required to be trained in the use of AEDs.

5. T F Chest pain is generally the main symptom of an acute MI in people over the age of 70.

6. T F Normal saline and Ringer's lactate are the IV fluids most often used during a code.

7. T F The crash cart and defibrillator are generally checked by nursing staff every shift.

8. T F Lethal dysrhythmias include A fib, V fib, idioventricular rhythm, and bradycardia.

9. T F Classic bradycardia is defined as any rhythm slow enough to cause hemodynamic compromise.

10. T F Electrical arcing can occur when nitroglycerin patches or paste are present during defibrillation.

Multiple Choice

1. Mrs. Saunders, a 76-year-old patient on your skilled nursing unit, is 8 days post–hip replacement. After report, you find her unresponsive, with no respirations and no pulse. She has no advance directive. Your action should be:

   a. Call a code from her bedside phone, call her family, and hold her hand while you wait for help.
   b. Get the crash cart, intubate her, and begin ventilation at 18 breaths /min.
   c. Use her bedside phone to activate the code team, yell for help, then begin mouth-to-mask ventilation and ask a coworker to begin chest compressions.
   d. Yell for help, send someone to call the physician, and then check the chart before beginning resuscitation procedures.

2. When the code team arrives, the quick look shows Mrs. Saunders is in ventricular fibrillation. You should prepare for:

   a. administration of vasoactive drugs.
   b. defibrillation.
   c. external pacing.
   d. synchronous cardioversion.

3. The code team is having difficulty gaining IV access and must use the endotracheal tube to deliver medications. Which ones can be administered via the ETT?

   a. Atropine, epinephrine, lidocaine
   b. Atropine, lidocaine, nitroglycerin
   c. Lidocaine, magnesium, verapamil
   d. Lidocaine, dopamine, furosemide

4. During the code, your intubated patient should be ventilated:

   a. after every fifth chest compression.
   b. asynchronously 12–15 times per minute.
   c. asynchronously 18–22 times per minute.
   d. during the fifth chest compression.

5. Your patient has a heart rate of 90–100 beats per minute and no visible P waves. Your initial response is to:

   a. call the physician to ask for orders for lidocaine.
   b. defibrillate immediately.
   c. call the physician to ask for orders for atropine.
   d. assess patient and perform a 12-lead ECG to diagnose rhythm.

6. Mr. Jones, 70, was admitted because of syncopal episodes. You find him in his room with no pulse or respirations. A code has been called, and ABGs were drawn before resuscitation was under way. You expect the blood gases to indicate:

   a. acidosis.
   b. alkalosis.
   c. compensated metabolic acidosis.
   d. normal range for his age.

7. The primary indication for use of adenosine is:

   a. sustained wide-complex SVT.
   b. sustained narrow-complex SVT.
   c. symptomatic bradycardia.
   d. sustained junctional tachycardia.

8. Beta-adrenergic receptor stimulation results in:

   a. bronchoconstriction.
   b. increased heart rate.
   c. negative chronotropism.
   d. negative inotropism.

9. Which statement best describes the effect of dopamine when used at low dosages (1–2 mcg/kg/min)?

   a. It has a negative inotropic effect, decreasing myocardial oxygen demand.
   b. It increases renal blood flow, thereby increasing urine output.
   c. It increases systolic BP and systemic vascular resistance.
   d. It suppresses junctional and ventricular ectopic beats.

10. Your patient is complaining of an intense headache and appears flushed within one minute after medication administration. What drug has he most likely been given?

    a. Adenosine
    b. Digoxin
    c. Lidocaine
    d. Nitroglycerin

Matching—Pharmacology

1. _____ Oxygen

2. _____ Atropine

3. _____ Epinephrine

4. _____ Lidocaine

5. _____ Procainamide

6. _____ Adenosine

7. _____ Bretylium

8. _____ Verapamil

9. _____ Diltiazem

10. _____ Dopamine

11. _____ Magnesium

12. _____ Sodium bicarbonate

13. _____ Calcium chloride

14. _____ Morphine

15. _____ Amiodarone

a. Used to treat underlying hypocalcemia, hyperkalemia, or calcium channel blocker toxicity

b. Can cause necrosis and sloughing of tissue if it infiltrates

c. Beneficial in treating prior metabolic acidosis, hyperkalemia, or overdose of tricyclic antidepressants or phenobarbitol

d. Increases heart rate by decreasing vagal tone

e. Initial drug of choice for SVT

f. Used in pulmonary edema to increase venous capacitance and decrease systemic vascular resistance; also used to treat ischemic chest pain.

g. Second-line antidysrhythmic; causes significant postural hypotension

h. Reduces rates of dysrhythmias and sudden cardiac death in patients with recent MI or CHF

i. Improves tissue oxygenation; treats hypoxemia resulting from inadequate gas exchange and/or inadequate CO

j. Drug of choice for ventricular ectopy; overdose causes lethargy, confusion, tinnitis, and paresthesias

k. Calcium channel blocker that slows heart rate but is not first choice

l. Potent vasoconstrictor; increases systemic vascular resistance, arterial BP; increases HR, myocardial oxygen demand

m. Treats ventricular ectopy and VT uncontrolled by lidocaine

n. Treatment of choice for torsades de pointes; essential for enzyme reactions and function of sodium-potassium pump

o. Useful in slowing rapid ventricular rates in A fib or A flutter

p. Different effects are obtained according to dosage

q. Must be administered slowly to prevent a decrease in HR

PERSONALIZE IT!!

❖ Your unit's crash cart and defibrillator must be checked by nursing staff every 24 hours. Volunteer to be trained for this and do it frequently to familiarize yourself with the contents and equipment.

❖ Current research indicates that families benefit from varying degrees of exposure to the code experience. Find, read, and share a research article on this topic.

❖ Ask your supervisor whether there are opportunities for you to participate in a "mock code." If not, investigate the possibility of initiating this exercise for interested nurses and interdisciplinary team members.

CROSSWORD PUZZLE

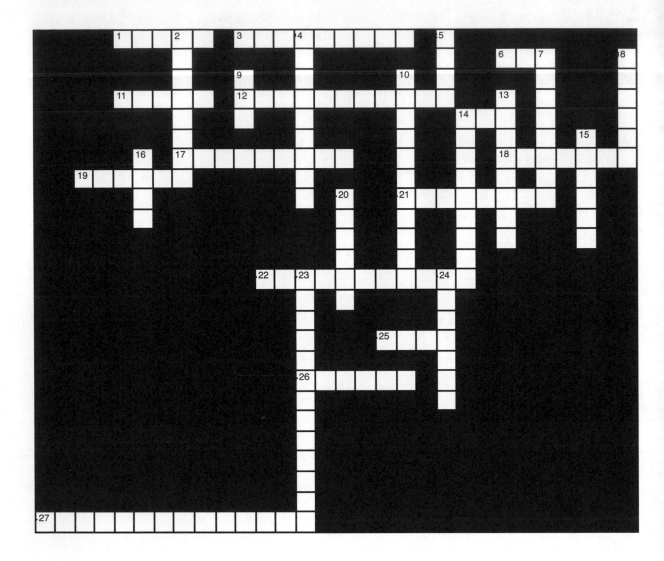

Across

1. Word shouted by person performing defibrillation to ensure that no one is touching the patient.
3. The second step of CPR is to look for, listen to, and feel for _____.
6. Abbreviation for device used to provide early defibrillation at the scene of a cardiac arrest.
11. Second nurse in a code coordinates the "_____ cart."
12. Drug that increases systemic vascular resistance, blood pressure, and heart rate.
14. One-person CPR is fifteen compressions of the chest to _____ breaths.
17. Drug of choice for VT, PVCs, and VF, but NEVER FOR BRADYCARDIA!
18. Nurse who should be available to relate information to the director of the code.
19. Preferred "normal" intravenous solution used during resuscitation efforts.
21. Drug that increases the heart rate by decreasing vagal tone.
22. Sodium _____ is the drug used to reverse an acidotic state; rarely used.
25. Abbreviation for Advanced Cardiac Life Support.
26. Brain damage may occur in 4 to 6 minutes if the brain does not receive enough _____.
27. The "D" in ABCDs of the primary survey.

Down

2. Absence of electrical activity of the heart.
4. Initial drug of choice for supraventricular dysrhythmias.
5. Emergency situations requiring life-saving resuscitation and interventions.
7. Drug given by infusion to increase blood pressure.
8. The first assessment after asking, "Are you okay?"
9. Abbreviation for dysrhythmia in which a rhythm is present on the monitor but no pulse is palpated.
10. Assessed by determining the presence of a pulse.
13. Analgesic used in the treatment of ischemic chest pain.
14. Accumulation of fluid in the pericardial sac.
15. Transcutaneous cardiac _____ is used to treat symptomatic bradycardia and asystole.
16. If a pulse is present, the nurse provides one breath every _____ seconds.
20. Oxygen is delivered through a bag-valve-mask device at 15 _____ per minute.
23. Process of synchronizing electrical energy on the R wave to disrupt a fast rhythm.
24. Pneumothorax that occurs when air enters the pleural space but cannot escape.

CONCEPT MAP

PEA refers to the absence of a detectable pulse and the presence of some type of electrical activity. It is often associated with clinical conditions that can be reversed if they are identified early and treated appropriately. Fill in the remainder of the chart as illustrated with the etiology of hypovolemia.

Possible Etiology	Data Needed/Clues	Management
Hypovolemia	History; flat neck veins	Volume infusion

Chapter 8

SHOCK

LEARNING OUTCOMES

- Define *shock*.
- Correlate the four classifications of shock to their pathophysiology.
- Discuss the progression of shock through the three stages.
- Identify assessment findings related to the classification and stage of shock.
- Identify definitive and supportive interventions related to the classification and stage of shock.
- Develop an individualized plan of care that includes nursing diagnosis, expected outcomes, and multidisciplinary interventions.

TERMINOLOGY

- anaerobic metabolism
- anaphylactic shock
- cardiogenic shock
- catecholamines
- colloid
- crystalloid
- disseminated intravascular coagulation (DIC)
- distributive shock
- fluid challenge
- hypovolemic shock
- intraaortic balloon pump (IABP)
- leukopenia
- microcirculation
- multiple organ failure
- neurogenic shock
- pneumatic antishock garment (PASG)
- septic shock
- systemic vascular resistance (SVR)
- third spacing

KEY POINTS

❖ Shock is a "clinical syndrome" affecting all body systems. There are different causes of shock, but two common characteristics exist in all cases. These are poor tissue perfusion and impaired cellular metabolism. Shock is classified into four categories, dependent on underlying causes. The four classifications and their pathophysiological mechanisms are as follows:

- Hypovolemic shock is characterized by a depletion of blood volume resulting in inadequate transport of oxygen and nutrients to tissues. Severity depends on volume loss, the patient's age, and presence of pre-existing conditions. Hypovolemic shock may be caused by external or internal volume deficits of blood, plasma, or body fluids.

  - External volume deficits may occur postpartum, after traumatic injury or surgery, or as a result of coagulation alterations. The most common cause of hypovolemic shock is hemorrhage.

  - Internal volume deficits may be caused by third space sequestration (e.g. ascites, peritonitis, edema), fluid leakage into the intestinal lumen (e.g. intestinal obstruction), or by internal hemorrhage (e.g., in patients with ruptured liver spleen, hemothorax, etc.)

  - Volume loss leads to decreased preload, decreased cardiac output, hypotension, decreased tissue perfusion, and impaired cellular metabolism.

  - Review of the definitions of cardiac dynamics terminology: *Preload* is the pressure in the ventricles as they fill. *Afterload* is the pressure the heart must overcome to effectively empty the ventricles.

- Cardiogenic shock occurs as a result of the failure of the heart to pump effectively. Pathophysiological sequences include a decrease in myocardial contractility (thus a decrease in stroke volume or the amount of blood ejected each minute), decreased cardiac output, hypotension, decreased tissue perfusion, and impaired cellular metabolism.

  - Most cardiac causes of cardiogenic shock are as a result of acute MI.

  - Other causes result from ineffective myocardial cell function such as dysrhythmias, cardiomyopathy, myocarditis, metabolic derangement, valvular disease, structural disorders, and vitamin deficiencies.

- Obstructive shock occurs as a result of physical impairment or obstruction to adequate circulatory flow in the heart or great vessels. Pathophysiological mechanisms include increased right ventricular afterload (e.g., as a result of pulmonary emboli, pulmonary hypertension), impaired diastolic filling, (e.g., pericardial tamponade, tension pneumothorax, compression of great veins, or constrictive pericarditis), and increased left ventricular afterload (e.g., as a result of aortic dissection, systemic embolization, aortic stenosis).

  - Obstruction causes decreased ventricular filling, decreased cardiac output, hypotension, decreased tissue perfusion, and impaired cellular metabolism.

- Distributive shock (vasogenic shock) describes several different types of shock (neurogenic, anaphylactic, septic). The commonality is widespread vasodilation and a decrease in stroke volume, cardiac output, and blood pressure resulting in decreased tissue perfusion. This results in a relative hypovolemia, in that blood volume remains normal but because of massive vasodilation and peripheral resistance, the blood is abnormally distributed in the enlarged vascular space, resulting in decreased venous return. A brief summary of the different types of distributive shock follows:

- Neurogenic shock: A disturbance in the nervous system affects the vasomotor center of the medulla. This center functions to initiate sympathetic stimulation of nerve fibers down the spinal cord to the periphery where they innervate smooth muscles of blood vessels to cause vasoconstriction. When this process is impeded, vasodilation results. Some causes of neurogenic shock include diseases of the upper spinal cord, spinal anesthesia, and nervous system damage.

- Anaphylactic shock: Results from a severe allergic reaction. Antigens enter the body, attach to mast cells and basophils which contain histamine (a potent vasodilator). This causes vasodilation, increased capillary permeability, smooth muscle contraction, decreased blood pressure, and relative hypovolemia. Symptoms involve the skin, respiratory and GI tracts.

- Septic shock: Caused by systemic inflammatory response, resulting from an infective process. Severe sepsis and septic shock are the most common causes of death in the ICU with a mortality rate of 40%–80%. Nosocomial infections are a major cause of sepsis in the critically ill. As bacteria are destroyed, endotoxins are released into the blood stream, damaging tissues and altering cellular metabolism. This results in cellular hypoxia and a decrease in energy. Endotoxins also release histamine, which leads to hypotension, venous pooling and decreased venous return. Compensatory tachycardia results.

❖ Progression of Shock (Regardless of Type)

- Early, reversible, compensatory stage: The body attempts to compensate for sustained reduction in cardiac output through neural, endocrine, and chemical mechanisms in an attempt to maintain blood flow to vital organs and restore homeostasis. The systemic and microcirculations work together through vasoconstriction to increase venous return. Types of early compensation include:

    - Neural—baroreceptors, autonomic nervous system, catecholamines, shunting of blood

    - Endocrine—hypothalamus, anterior/posterior pituitary glands, adrenocorticotropic hormones, glucocorticoids, mineralcorticoids (aldosterone), juxtoglomerular apparatus, renin-angiotensin

    - Chemical—chemoreceptors stimulate hyperventilation, CO excretion, and respiratory alkalosis; causes vasoconstriction of cerebral blood vessels, cerebral hypoxia, and ischemia (negative effect)

- Intermediate/progressive stage: Further patient deterioration occurs when the cause of shock is not corrected and compensatory mechanisms do not work. Systemic and microcirculation no longer work together but function independently and in opposition with the systemic circulation continuing to vasoconstrict in an attempt to shunt blood to vital organs. The microcirculation exerts an opposite effect of dilation in order to obtain a blood supply for local tissue needs. Signs and symptoms affect all body systems. The patient responds poorly to fluid replacement alone and requires aggressive medical treatment.

- Refractory/irreversible stage: Prolonged, inadequate tissue perfusion, which is unresponsive to therapy and ultimately contributes to multiple organ failure and death. Severe tissue hypoxia, necrosis, cerebral ischemia, vasodilation, bradycardia, decreased BP and heart rate, and multisystem organ failure occur.

❖ Assessment Findings Related to Classification and Stage

- Cardiovascular system:

    - BP—Pulse pressure (difference between systolic and diastolic pressures) continues to narrow. May need to assess BP by palpation or alternative means in later stages.

    - Pulses—Evaluate all pulses. Tachycardia may occur as an attempt to increase perfusion but can result in decreased cardiac output. In the irreversible stage, bradycardia develops related to metabolic acidosis and release of myocardial depressant factor.

    - Heart sounds—Abnormal heart sounds S_3 and S_4 are heard with cardiogenic shock.

    - Neck veins—Distended in cardiogenic and obstructive shock; flat in hypovolemic shock.

    - Capillary refill—Delay indicates peripheral vasoconstriction.

    - Right atrial pressure—Decreased in hypovolemic shock, and increased in cardiogenic and obstructive shock.

    - Hemodynamic monitoring

        - Preload (fluid balance)—RAP (right atrial pressure); PCWP (pulmonary capillary wedge pressure) or left atrial pressure.

        - Afterload (vascular resistance)—SVR (systemic vascular resistance); PVR (pulmonary vascular resistance)

        - Cardiac output and cardiac index provide information on contractile force and how the heart is handling the cell's demands for nutrients.

        - SVO_2 (mixed venous oxygen saturation) evaluates whether or not the oxygen supply is meeting the tissue needs.

- Respiratory system: In the early stages of shock the body attempts to compensate for metabolic acidosis. Chemoreceptors stimulate the medulla with an increase in rate and depth of respiration. As shock continues, respiratory muscles weaken due to metabolic waste build-up leading to shallow breathing, poor air exchange, and acute respiratory distress.

- Renal system: Urine output less than 30 ml/hr reflects shock. Kidneys compensate, decreasing excreted fluids and concentrating urine. Renin-angiotensin mechanism facilitates release of aldosterone, with retention of sodium and reabsorption of water further decreasing urinary output. With progression of shock, there is an increase in Na, BUN and creatinine levels.

- GI system: Initial response to shock is decreased flow to the "non-essential" GI organs, resulting in slowed intestinal activity, decreased bowel sounds, distention, nausea, and constipation. With progression, there is decreased motility, increased permeability of the tract lining leading to paralytic ileus, ulceration, and damaged lining. The damage allows bacteria to enter the systemic circulation, thus an increased risk of infection. There is hypoperfusion of the liver and alterations in liver enzymes. With progression there is a decreased production of clotting factors, and the liver will not detoxify drugs or neutralize microorganisms.

- Hematologic system: In the early stages, blood cells and flow become sluggish and with decreased perfusion, microemboli are formed. Leukopenia results because of compensatory depletion of the WBCs, thus increasing susceptibility to infection. With the decrease in clotting factor formation by the liver, risk of disseminated intravascular coagulation (DIC) increases.

- Skin and mucous membranes: Evaluate color, temp, texture, turgor, and moisture levels. Changes in different types of shock: (1) Septic—moist, flushed, warm; (2) Hypovolemic or cardiogenic—pale, cool, moist, mucous membranes dry; (3) Anaphylactic—urticaria and pruritus; (4) Toxic shock syndrome—red macular rash, desquamation of skin.

  - Cyanosis (central or peripheral) is a late sign of shock.

- Musculoskeletal system: Generalized weakness and fatigue is caused by increased lactate levels with progression to myoglobinemia due to breakdown of skeletal muscle.

- Neurological system: Restlessness, irritability, and apprehension occur, progressing to listlessness, agitation, apathy, confusion. There is a decreased response to painful stimuli in the progressive stage, leading to unconsciousness, absent reflexes, and dilated pupils with absent response to light.

❖ Definitive and Supportive Interventions

- Treatment is aimed at correcting or reversing the cause of alteration in circulation. Care includes the following: fluid, pharmacological, mechanical therapies to maintain tissue perfusion, as well as interventions to increase oxygen delivery.

- Hypovolemic, or distributive, shock requires the administration of IV fluids. Choice of fluid, rate and volume depend on the type of loss and concurrent medical problems. Crystalloids, colloids, blood, and blood products are used alone or in combination to restore intravascular volume.

- Crystalloids (e.g., lactated Ringer's or 0.9% normal saline) are used initially (3 ml of crystalloid to replace each 1 ml of blood loss).

- Colloids may be given instead (these contain protein, increase osmotic pressure, increase fluid volume, and expand plasma volume). Types of colloids: albumin, plasmanate or synthetic types.

- Dangers of large volumes of crystalloids include hemodilution of RBCs and plasma proteins with impairment of oxygen delivery to the cells, decrease in colloidal osmotic pressure, and an increased risk of pulmonary edema. Pulmonary edema is also a complication of colloid administration.

- Blood and blood products—whole blood, packed RBCs, washed RBCs, fresh frozen plasma, and platelets are given for the treatment of major blood loss.

- Blood and blood products are given until the Hgb is greater than or equal to 10g/dl. Types of adverse reactions to blood transfusions include circulatory overload, hemolysis, allergy, hyperthermia, hypothermia, hyperkalemia, hypocalcemia. In the event of reaction, the infusion is stopped, tubing is disconnected from the access site, and the vein is kept open with 0.9% NS. Physician and lab are notified. All transfusion equipment is sent to the lab.

- Along with fluid administration, drugs that increase preload are used as adjunctive therapy for distributive shock (e.g., vasopressors, such as epinephrine and norepinephrine.) Afterload is low in distributive shock; drugs that increase afterload may be given (e.g., epinephrine).

- Cardiogenic shock is managed primarily with pharmacological agents, which act through manipulation of cardiac dynamics.

- Types of drugs (see Table 8-11):

  - Positive inotropic agents (dopamine, dobutamine, norepinephrine, amrinone)

  - Drugs to reduce preload (nitroprusside, diuretics, nitrates, nitroglycerin, morphine)

- Drugs to reduce afterload (nitroprusside and nitroglycerin)

- Drugs that alter heart rate (chronotropic and antidysrhythmic drugs)

❖ Mechanical Management

- Management is aimed at restoration of perfusion to cells and includes the following:

  - Intraaortic balloon pump (IABP)—most often used in cardiogenic shock

  - Ventricular assist device—inserted to assume cardiac pumping function, as a temporary measure to support a failing ventricle in cardiogenic shock

  - Pneumatic antishock garment (PASG)—may be used as a temporary measure to provide circulatory assistance in hypovolemic shock

❖ Nursing Interventions

- Interventions are aimed at support of tissue perfusion and maintenance of organ function and include the following:

  - Maintain a patent airway and intravenous access.

  - Position patient using slight elevation of lower extremities.

  - Maintain body temperature and skin integrity.

  - Administer fluids as ordered and evaluate response.

  - Assess the status of cardiopulmonary, neurological, and GI systems.

  - Assess serial serum and urine values (H&H, PT, PTT, fibrin, fibrinogen, platelets, ABGs, chemistry profile, lactate, blood cultures).

  - Assess pain levels and administer meds as prescribed.

  - Provide adequate nutritional and psychological support.

❖ Nursing Diagnosis

- Altered tissue perfusion related to:

  - Decreased blood volume

  - Decreased myocardial contractility

  - Impaired circulatory blood flow

  - Widespread vasodilation secondary to hypovolemic, cardiogenic, obstructive, or distributive shock

❖ Patient Outcomes

- Patient will have improved tissue perfusion. Specific outcomes: alertness, orientation, normotension, warmth, dry skin, adequate urine output, hemodynamic and lab values within normal limits, absence of infection, and intact skin.

REVIEW QUESTIONS

True/False

1. T F   One of the effects shock has on the body is that the cells undergo aerobic metabolism, which leads to the development of lactic acidosis.

2. T F   The patient in shock is best positioned in the Trendelenburg position, in order to increase venous return without compromising ventilatory status.

3. T F   The nurse would expect to find the following hemodynamic alterations in a patient with cardiogenic shock: decreased cardiac output, increased pulmonary capillary wedge pressure, increased systemic vascular resistance.

4. T F   Systemic inflammatory response syndrome (SIRS) is the initial stage of progressive deterioration in anaphylactic shock.

5. T F   When assessing the patient's response to a fluid challenge, the nurse describes the patient as having a transient response to the initial fluid administration. The nurse can accurately conclude that the patient has remained hemodynamically normal and that fluids can be slowed to a maintenance rate.

6. T F   Current recommendations for the administration of crystalloids are to administer an initial rapid fluid bolus of 1–2 liters for an adult.

7. T F   Colloids contain proteins, increase osmotic pressure and expand plasma volume. Compared with crystalloids, smaller volumes of colloids are given.

8. T F   One of the major side effects of administration of packed red blood cells is volume overload.

9. T F   Positive inotropic agents such as dopamine are given to increase the contractile force of the heart and are used in the management of hypovolemic shock.

10. T F   Hematocrit and hemoglobin are decreased in hypovolemic shock caused by hemorrhage.

Multiple Choice

1. The portion of the vascular bed most significant for cell survival is:

   a. pulmonary circulation.
   b. arteriole.
   c. microcirculation.
   d. systemic circulation.

2. The majority of cases of cardiogenic shock are caused by:

   a. pancreatitis.
   b. anaphylaxis.
   c. acute myocardial infarction (AMI).
   d. gastrointestinal (GI) bleed.

3. When neurogenic shock occurs, interruption in sympathetic nerve impulses causes:

   a. hypertension.
   b. vasodilation.
   c. hyperventilation.
   d. bradycardia.

4. Vasodilation occurring in distributive shock results in:

   a. decreased heart rate.
   b. increased venous return.
   c. decreased preload.
   d. increased afterload.

5. The substances released from cellular breakdown mediated by the antigen-antibody reaction cause:

   a. hypovolemia.
   b. increased capillary permeability.
   c. vasoconstriction.
   d. relaxation of smooth muscle.

6. In the initial stage of shock, decreased cardiac output results in:

   a. increased sympathetic stimulation.
   b. increased parasympathetic stimulation.
   c. increased vagal stimulation.
   d. increased urine output.

7. In response to decreased renal perfusion, the juxtaglomerular apparatus releases:

   a. angiotensin.
   b. renin.
   c. aldosterone.
   d. antidiuretic hormone (ADH).

8. Blood pooling in the capillary bed and arterial blood pressure too low to support perfusion of vital organs causes:

   a. CNS disturbances.
   b. pancreatitis.
   c. pneumonia.
   d. multisystem organ failure (MOF).

9. The first system to be affected by changes in cellular perfusion is the:

   a. cardiovascular system.
   b. central nervous system.
   c. respiratory system.
   d. gastrointestinal system.

10. The most sensitive method of assessing oxygenation in shock is:

    a. pulse oximetry.
    b. ABGs.
    c. auscultation.
    d. capillary refill.

Matching—Key Terms

1. _____ IABP

2. _____ Respiratory alkalosis

3. _____ Septic shock

4. _____ Acute respiratory distress syndrome

5. _____ Anaerobic metabolism

6. _____ Relative hypovolemia

7. _____ Lactated Ringer's solution

8. _____ Lactate levels

9. _____ Cardiogenic shock

10. _____ Angiotensin II

a. Vessels dilate while blood volume remains constant

b. A complication of shock associated with hypoperfusion and pulmonary hypotension

c. Isotonic crystalloid used in the initial resuscitation from shock as a result of hemorrhage

d. One of the most difficult types of shock to treat with a mortality rate of 75%–85%

e. The most common cause of death in ICUs with a mortality rate of 40%–80%

f. A potent vasoconstrictor that increases blood pressure and improves venous return

g. Condition occurring in the compensatory stage of shock associated with hyperventilation

h. Cells convert to this type of metabolism in response to cellular hypoxia

i. A marker of anaerobic metabolism (elevated levels indicate significant hypoperfusion)

j. Most often used in cardiogenic shock to increase coronary artery perfusion and reduce afterload

PERSONALIZE IT!!

❖ Administering blood and blood products is a task with great potential for error and serious injury to the patient. Familiarize yourself with your organization's policy regarding administration of blood and blood products. Observe nurses during the process of checking blood products prior to administration.

❖ The early post-surgical period is a time to be especially alert for hypovolemic shock. What measures can you employ in your assessments to ensure early detection of hypovolemia?

CROSSWORD PUZZLE

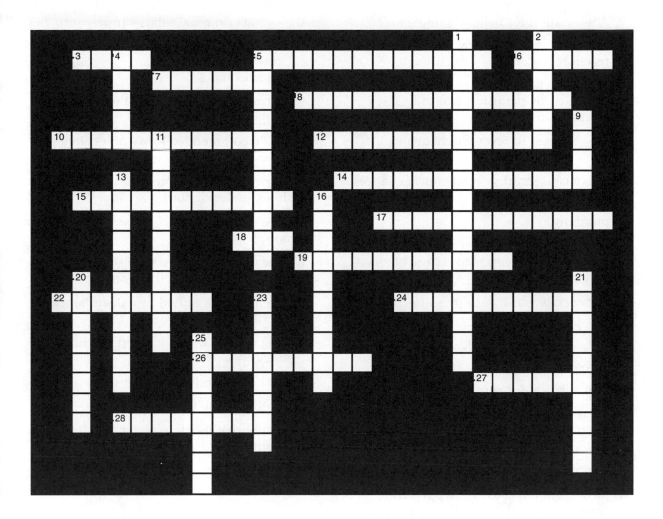

Across

3. Abbreviation for balloon pump.

5. Type of shock caused by a severe allergic reaction.

6. Clinical syndrome characterized by inadequate tissue perfusion and cellular metabolism alteration.

7. _____ is used to reverse ischemia to myocytes.

8. Nerve cells sensitive to chemical changes.

10. Type of shock caused by ineffective heart pumping.

12. Stage of shock in which activation of mechanisms attempts to restore blood volume.

14. Nerve cells sensitive to pressure changes.

15. .9% normal saline is a _____.

17. Type of shock caused by widespread vasodilation.

18. Abbreviation for ventricular assist device.

19. Stage of shock in which systemic and microcirculation oppose vasoconstriction.

22. _____ contain proteins that increase osmotic pressure.

24. Most common cause of hypovolemic shock.

26. This type of compensation involves message relay to the hypothalamus.

27. Type of shock caused by systemic inflammatory syndrome; often associated with infection.

28. _____ inotropic agents increase contractile force of the heart.

Down

1. _____ act on renal tubules to reabsorb Na^+, thus increasing volume.

2. Urine output of less than _____ ml/hour indicates shock.

4. Special Y-set tubing is used to administer _____.

5. Area recommended for IV access in shock patient.

9. Major respiratory complication related to shock (abbreviation).

11. Type of shock caused by vessel compression.

13. Type of shock caused by insufficient amount of blood in the vessels.

16. Type of shock caused by a disturbance in the CNS.

20. Drug used to increase blood pressure in shock.

21. Final and terminal stage of shock.

23. Another name for norepinephrine.

25. Distributive shock results in _____ hypovolemia.

CONCEPT MAP

Comprehensive Data Map

Complete a comprehensive data map for Mr. B., an 82-year-old man brought into the local emergency department in a confused and disoriented state. Mr. B. is diabetic and has an open ulcer on his right great toe draining purulent fluid. His vital signs include the following: temp 103.9° F, BP 66/42, HR 112, respiratory rate 40 and shallow.

Client Medical Diagnosis

Laboratory Studies

Pertinent History

Predisposing Factors of the Diagnosis

Diagnostic Studies

Prioritized Problem List

Supportive Measures

Definitive Treatment
(possible prescribed meds, treatments, IV fluids)

Chapter 9

CARDIAC ALTERATIONS

LEARNING OUTCOMES

- Contrast the pathological cause and effect mechanisms that produce acute cardiac disturbances.
- Discuss the nursing care responsibilities related to the cardiac patient.
- Compare and contrast pharmacological, operative, and electrical modalities used in treatment of cardiac disease.
- Identify specific nursing interventions designed to prevent secondary occurrences or to minimize complications of cardiac patients.
- Develop a research-related care plan for the acutely ill cardiac patient.

TERMINOLOGY

- angina
- angioplasty
- antidysrhythmics
- atheroma
- automaticity
- autotransfusion
- baroreceptors
- cardiac enzymes
- cardiac reserve
- chemoreceptors
- conductivity
- congestive heart failure (CHF)
- coronary artery bypass graft (CABG)

- coronary artery disease (CAD)
- endocarditis
- endocardium
- epicardium
- excitability
- hyperlipidemia
- insufficiency
- intraaortic balloon pump (IABP)
- lipoproteins
- murmur
- myocardial infarction (MI)
- myocardium
- nitrates

- palpitations
- pericarditis
- pulmonary edema
- Q wave versus non-Q wave MI
- rhythmicity
- S_1
- S_2
- S_3
- S_4
- stent
- stroke volume (SV)
- troponin
- vasodilators

91

KEY POINTS

❖ Review of Normal Cardiac Structure and Function

- The heart muscle has three layers: the outer epicardium, the middle muscular myocardium, and the inner endothelial endocardium.

- The five basic properties of cardiac muscle are contractility, rhythmicity, conductivity, automaticity, and excitability.

- The right atrium receives deoxygenated blood via the superior and inferior venae cavae.

- Blood flows through the tricuspid valve to the right ventricle, then through the pulmonic valve to the pulmonary artery, delivering it to the lungs for oxygen and carbon dioxide exchange.

- Pulmonary veins deliver the oxygenated blood to the left atrium, through the mitral valve to the left ventricle, then through the aortic valve into the aorta for systemic circulation.

- The tricuspid and mitral valves are atrioventricular or AV valves; they are anchored by chordae tendineae to the papillary muscles on the ventricular floor. The pulmonic and aortic valves are referred to as semilunar valves, which open and close passively as a result of changing pressures.

❖ Heart Sounds

- S_1 ("lubb") indicates closure of mitral and tricuspid valves at the beginning of ventricular systole.

- S_2 ("dubb") indicates closure of aortic and pulmonic valves at the beginning of ventricular diastole.

- S_3 ("lubb-dubb-a") is normal in children; often an early indicator of CHF in adults; occurs immediately after S_2.

- S_4 ("te-lubb-dubb") is a forceful atrial contraction; often occurs after MI; precedes S_1.

- In severe heart failure, all four produce "gallop" – "te-lubb-dubb-a".

❖ Autonomic Control

- Sympathetic nervous system (SNS) releases norepinephrine.

- Alpha-adrenergic effects = vasoconstriction.

- Beta-adrenergic effects = + chronotrope, + inotrope, + dromotrope.

- Parasympathetic nervous system (PNS) releases acetylcholine through stimulation of the vagus nerve; decreases sinus node discharge and slows AV conduction.

❖ Chemoreceptors

- Chemoreceptors control vasoconstriction and vasodilation in response to arterial gas partial pressures. Baroreceptors are sensitive to stretch and pressure.

❖ Coronary Artery Disease (CAD)

- CAD is the progressive narrowing of one or more coronary arteries by atherosclerosis; injury occurs when internal diameter of the vessel is reduced by 50% to 70%.

- Atherosclerosis begins with injury to the intima, resulting in platelet aggregation, monocyte migration, and formation of a fatty streak. Lipid-rich "foam cells" develop, then progress to a fibrous plaque or atheroma.

- Platelet-derived growth factor (PDGF) stimulates smooth cell migration into the intima, forming the atheroma, which becomes a fibrous cap. The cap can rupture, producing a thrombus that may occlude a coronary artery.

- Platelet changes occur in three steps: (1) adhesion (at site of injury); (2) activation (GpIIb/IIIa receptors bind with von Willebrand's factor and fibrinogen), and (3) aggregation with one another. These steps produce a fast-growing thrombus that compromises blood flow.

- Major risk factors for CAD: age (men over 45, women over 55), family history, high blood cholesterol (> 200 mg/dl), smoking, hypertension, diabetes, obesity/overweight, and physical inactivity.

  - Secondary risk factors are being investigated: stress, alcohol, and the role of estrogen.

- Assessment for CAD includes a thorough history of childhood and recent illnesses, as well as any record of rheumatic fever, diabetes mellitus, hypertension, asthma, CVA, or renal disease. Medications are listed, including use of Viagra and OTC drugs. Psychosocial history facilitates discharge planning.

- For assessing any patient with chest pain, use this helpful mnemonic: **PQRST**—**P**rovocation, **Q**uality, **R**egion/**R**adiation, **S**everity, and **T**iming/**T**reatment.

- Diagnostic studies for CAD:

  - Noninvasive tests—12-lead ECG, Holter monitor, exercise tolerance (stress) tests, chest x-ray, magnetic resonance imaging (MRI), and echocardiogram.

  - Invasive tests—transesophageal echocardiogram (TEE), radioisotope contrast studies (minimally invasive), and cardiac catheterization/arteriography.

- Lab tests—serum electrolytes (hypokalemia is a common abnormality) and serum enzymes:

  - Creatinine kinase (CK)—not specific for cardiac damage; increases within 2–6 hours of AMI; peaks in 18–36 hours.

  - CK-MB—specific for cardiac muscle damage; rises in 4–18 hours; peaks in 18–24 hours; serial CK and CK-MBs are run at onset, 8, 16, and 24 hours.

  - Cardiac troponin I or T—rises as early as 1 hour after damage; more specific than CK-MB at 7–14 hour point.

  - Myoglobin: released in serum 30–60 minutes after AMI.

- Medical management:

  - Risk factor modification includes a low-fat, low-cholesterol diet, exercise, weight control, smoking cessation, and control of diabetes and hypertension. Lipid-lowering drugs are used if a six-month modification period does not lower LDL levels.

    - Statins (HMG-CoA reductase inhibitors)—most effective but expensive; slow production of cholesterol and increase liver's ability to remove LDL from the body (lovastatin, pravastatin, simvastatin).

    - Bile acid resins—combine with cholesterol-containing bile acids to form insoluble complex that is eliminated through feces.

- Nicotinic acid (niacin)—high doses reduce total cholesterol, LDL, and triglycerides; OTC but must be under medical supervision.

- Gemfibrozil targets triglycerides; produces GI side effects.

- Platelet adhesion and aggregation inhibitors are used for long-term therapy for angina, transient ischemic attacks, and valve replacements. Daily aspirin therapy or agents such as dipyridamole, ticlopidine, and clopidrogrel may be prescribed.

- Expected patient outcomes: Verbalize absence or relief of pain, feel less anxiety, understand the disease process, and adhere to behaviors that are beneficial to health

❖ Angina

- Angina is an acute intermittent chest pain syndrome caused by imbalance between myocardial oxygen demand and supply and resultant myocardial ischemia. CAD and coronary artery spasm are common etiologies.

- Types of angina:

  - Stable angina occurs with exertion and is relieved by rest.

  - Unstable angina is an acute coronary syndrome involving partial blockage by a thrombus; pain is more severe, is not relieved by rest, and requires more frequent nitroglycerin therapy. Increased risk exists for MI.

  - Variant (Prinzmetal's) angina occurs at rest, as a result of coronary artery spasm; can lead to acute MI even without CAD.

- Diagnostics include thorough history, physical exam, and labs (H&H, cardiac enzymes, cholesterol levels, resting and event ECG, stress test, and angiography).

- Pharmacological management includes nitrates, beta-blockers, calcium channel blockers, and aspirin.

  - Patient education on use of nitrates (NTG):

    - Keep tablets readily available.

    - Take a tablet before strenuous activity.

    - If chest pain occurs, stop activity, sit down, and breathe. Take 1 NTG tablet sublingually. Repeat if needed in 5 minutes, up to total of 3 tablets. If pain persists, dial 911.

    - Store NTG tablets in the original dark bottle. Get a new supply every six months.

    - Avoid caffeine.

  - Beta-blockers decrease HR, BP, and cardiac contractility.

  - Calcium channel blockers inhibit the flow of calcium ions across cellular membranes, which increases myocardial blood flow and perfusion and thus decreases oxygen demand.

  - Taking 325 mg aspirin daily is a conservative treatment.

  - New treatments for unstable angina include GpIIb/IIIa inhibitors (abciximab, tirofiban, eptifibatide) and low molecular weight heparin (subcutaneously).

- Nursing interventions focus on maintenance of adequate CO, relief of pain and anxiety, and education that promotes self-care behaviors.

❖ Myocardial Infarction (MI)

- MI is caused by reduced blood flow to an area of the myocardium, resulting in significant and sustained oxygen deprivation to myocardial cells. Most infarcts occur in the left ventricle.

- MI evolves over a period of about three hours and is irreversible. Size of the infarct can be limited by early treatment (e.g., thrombolytics). "Time = muscle."

- Q wave MIs involve total occlusion of a coronary artery, secondary to a thrombus or ruptured plaque. ST segment elevation and elevated cardiac enzymes are seen. Thrombolytics are recommended.

- Non-Q wave MI usually results from partial occlusion. ST segment depression and elevated cardiac enzymes are seen. No Q wave develops.

- Assessment: Sudden, severe chest pain is the classic symptom (often described as crushing). Pain may radiate to arms, neck, or jaw. Skin may be cool, clammy, pale, and diaphoretic. NTG does not relieve this pain. Denial and an impending sense of doom are common. Symptoms for women are often atypical, and women are less likely to call 911; therefore, valuable treatment time is lost. Aspirin (162.5 mg) should be administered as soon as possible.

- Diagnostics: Symptoms, 12-lead ECG, and cardiac enzymes. ECG is the primary diagnostic criterion for acute MI. Lab data include CK, CK-MB; cardiac troponin T and I. Electrolytes should be checked, especially potassium. Bedside echocardiography may assist in diagnosis. Cardiac scanning helps identify infarct. Hemodynamic monitoring may be needed.

- Nursing interventions: Take a thorough history. Oxygen, NTG, and morphine are generally ordered. Monitor rhythm, BP, hemodynamics, and heart and lung sounds constantly. Maintain a calm, quiet environment and pay attention to psychosocial needs.

- Pharmacological treatment:

  - Initial pain is treated with IV morphine sulfate. Monitor for respiratory depression and hypotension. Nitroglycerin also reduces pain by increasing perfusion through vasodilation.

  - Thrombolytic therapy—Goal is to dissolve the occluding lesion and restore blood flow. Must be given within first 6 hours. Used in Q-wave MI.

  - Platelet aggregation inhibitors—Aspirin (162.5 mg) is given immediately. GpIIb/IIIa inhibitors are used in non-Q wave MI and are being used in combination with thrombolytics in trials of AMI treatment.

  - Use of heparin (anticoagulant) is controversial. Low molecular weight heparin is preferred.

  - Other medications frequently used in treatment of AMI include beta blockers (to decrease HR, BP, and myocardial O_2 consumption); nitrates (for vasodilation); and ACE inhibitors (to reduce ventricular remodeling).

- Knowledge deficit:

  - For the patient who survives MI and his or her family, education is essential. Understanding the purpose of various medications and possible side effects will promote compliance with the therapeutic regimen. Lifestyle changes (diet, weight, smoking cessation), cardiac rehabilitation, spiritual growth, and advance directives are a few of the areas to be addressed.

❖ Treatments for CAD and AMI

- Some hospitals perform emergent percutaneous intervention (PCI), including percutaneous transluminal coronary angioplasty (PTCA), an arteriography procedure that compresses intracoronary plaque, used especially in single-vessel disease. Patient must be a candidate for CABG in case of complications.

- Intracoronary stents are tubes implanted at the site of stenosis to provide structural support. Anticoagulation therapy is necessary after placement.

- Coronary artery bypass graft (CABG) is the replacement of blocked coronary artery or arteries with saphenous vein, internal mammary artery, or radial artery grafts. Drainage of postsurgical area is by means of chest and mediastinal tubes. NEVER CLAMP the chest tube; this could cause a tension pneumothorax.

- Minimally invasive coronary artery surgery (MIDCAB) avoids use of heart-lung machine and is easier on the patient.

- Transmyocardial revascularization (TMR) is accomplished by laser penetrations through damaged tissue, thus allowing blood flow to the infarcted areas. Relief of symptoms occurs over time.

❖ Management of Dysrhythmias

- Permanent pacemakers may be required for recurrent bradycardia or tachydysrhythmias.

  - The generator is inserted in the subcutaneous tissue of the upper chest; electrodes are usually placed tranvenously into the atria or ventricle.

  - Most pacemakers are multiprogrammable for rate, voltage, sensitivity, stimulus duration, and refractory periods.

  - Ventricular demand mode is commonly used.

  - Most are programmed to sense atrial or ventricular activity and respond with an appropriate stimulus.

  - Most use lithium batteries, which last 8–10 years.

- Implantable cardioverter/defibrillator (ICD):

  - ICDs are appropriate for patients with life-threatening ventricular dysrhythmias unresponsive to other treatments. Most also have pacemaker capabilities (PCD).

  - Small generator is implanted (similar to pacemaker) and delivers high-energy shocks when programmed dysrhythmia is detected, or paces if needed.

  - Complications include infection, lead failure, and unauthentic shocks for SVTs.

❖ Congestive Heart Failure (CHF)

- CHF is the second most common post-MI complication and can also result from CAD and hypertension.

- Causes:

  - CHF results from the inability of either ventricle to pump blood adequately to the systemic circulation. Resultant fluid backup leads to pulmonary edema and/or systemic congestion. Gas exchange is impaired and cardiac output is decreased.

  - Systolic HF results from impaired pumping of the ventricle(s) or increased afterload.

  - Diastolic HF results from impaired filling of the ventricles.

- Right-sided failure is usually caused by left-sided failure but can also result from pulmonary disease or right ventricular infarct. The predominant feature is fluid retention.

- With left-sided failure, the predominant feature is dyspnea.

- Assessment:

  - Left-sided failure—anxiety, dyspnea, orthopnea, crackles and wheezes.

  - Right-sided failure—dependent edema, jugular venous distention, liver engorgement and splenomegaly.

  - SNS activity produces tachycardia, vasoconstriction, and increased contractility.

- Diagnostics: hemodynamic monitoring, ABGs, electrolytes, CBC (to detect anemia), chest x-ray, liver function tests.

- Treatment:

  1. Improve pump function with ACE inhibitors and diuretics, also digoxin and vasodilators.

  2. Reduce cardiac workload and O_2 consumption by reducing anxiety and scheduling rest periods.

  3. Use intraaortic balloon pump (in severe CHF).

  4. Optimize gas exchange with supplemental O_2, diuresis, fluid restriction, cautious IV therapy, and low-sodium diet.

- Complications include pulmonary edema and cardiogenic shock.

- Knowledge deficit: Frequent readmission can be prevented if patients understand the importance of fluid and sodium restrictions, adherence to medication regimen, daily weight monitoring, and recognition of increasing dyspnea, orthopnea, and edema as warning signs.

REVIEW QUESTIONS

True/False

1. **T F**   Coronary heart disease remains the leading cause of morbidity and mortality in the United States.

2. **T F**   Treatment of the patient with acute MI consists of maintaining adequate myocardial oxygenation and increasing myocardial workload.

3. **T F**   A complication of PTCA and coronary artery stent placement is reocclusion.

4. **T F**   The most common major complication of PTCA is hypotension.

5. **T F**   Cardiac tamponade is a life-threatening complication that may occur after CABG surgery.

6. **T F**   When a patient with a pacemaker experiences loss of capture, it means a spike and QRS are seen but no pulse is felt.

7. **T F**   Cardiac glycoside (digoxin) is effective over a wide therapeutic range.

8. **T F**   Following insertion of a transvenous pacemaker, the nurse should encourage full ROM of the affected shoulder.

9. **T F**   Side effects of nitrate therapy include headache, nausea, dizziness, and hypertension.

10. **T F**   The most common cause of right-sided heart failure is left-sided heart failure.

Multiple Choice

1. The three major coronary arteries are:

   a.   right anterior descending, left anterior descending, and right circumflex.
   b.   right anterior descending, left posterior ascending, and left circumflex.
   c.   left coronary artery, left artery descending, and left circumflex.
   d.   right coronary artery, left anterior descending, left circumflex.

2. The left circumflex artery supplies:

   a.   AV node, left atrium, posterior left ventricles.
   b.   posterior ventricular septum, entire posterior wall, left atrium.
   c.   posterior ventricular septum, part of left atrium, entire posterior wall.
   d.   posterosuperior ventricular septum, part of left atrium, posterior left ventricle.

3. A galloping heartbeat can be heard with the bell of the stethoscope at the fifth intercostal space in a patient with:

   a.   pericarditis.
   b.   overforceful atrial contraction.
   c.   post MI.
   d.   severely failing heart.

4. The following diagnostic studies are ordered for a patient with CAD. Which identifies valvular function, measures the chamber size, and evaluates cardiac disease progression?

   a. 12-lead ECG
   b. Cardiac catheterization
   c. Echocardiogram
   d. Radioisotope studies

5. The fastest rising cardiac enzymes are:

   a. CPK and MB.
   b. SGOT and LFT.
   c. SGPT and CPK.
   d. troponins and CK-MB.

6. Angina is a transient event; however, it may be a precursor to cell death from myocardial ischemia. The nurse's first action for a patient experiencing anginal chest pain is to:

   a. administer pain medication and intubate.
   b. administer pain medication and elevate head of bed.
   c. encourage patient to hyperventilate.
   d. provide O_2, position at rest, and offer NTG.

7. Which of the following is/are characteristic of unstable angina?

   a. A change in duration and frequency of the chest pain
   b. A change in precipitating factors for the chest pain
   c. A change in the quality of the chest pain
   d. All of the above

8. Chest tubes are removed when:

   a. lungs are reexpanded and negative pressure is reestablished.
   b. lungs are reexpanded and positive pressure is reestablished.
   c. pleural space is reexpanded.
   d. tension pneumothorax is identified.

9. Pulmonary edema is a life-threatening form of CHF. Treatments for this condition include:

   a. IV morphine, aminophylline, and bumetanide.
   b. IV morphine, cysophylline, and furosemide.
   c. IV pentobarbital, aminophylline, and furosemide.
   d. IV pentobarbital, cysophylline, and bumetanide.

10. A concern for a patient being treated for CHF is:

   a. decreasing PCWP.
   b. digitalis toxicity.
   c. nitrate poisoning.
   d. normovolemia.

11. If a post-MI patient has received thrombolytic therapy, what must be closely monitored during and for a period of time after the therapy?

    a. Bleeding at the IV site
    b. ECG pattern
    c. Level of consciousness
    d. All of the above

12. Which of the following would be expected in right-sided heart failure?

    a. Dependent edema and hepatosplenomegaly
    b. Jugular vein distention and decreased heart rate
    c. Orthopnea and crackles in lung bases
    d. Tachycardia and a prolonged QT segment

13. Which sound is often an early sign of congestive heart failure?

    a. S_1
    b. S_2
    c. S_3
    d. S_4

14. The most essential diagnostic test done before cardiac surgery is:

    a. 12-lead ECG
    b. Cardiac arteriography
    c. Holter monitoring
    d. Saphenous vein angiography

15. Which of the following is the most significant finding in an assessment of a patient experiencing chest pain? The pain:

    a. increases with inspiration.
    b. is relieved with one NTG tablet.
    c. is relieved with rest.
    d. lasts longer than 30 minutes.

16. Of the following, which would be inappropriate in the nursing care of a patient who has just undergone a PTCA?

    a. Ambulate the patient within the first 2 hours.
    b. Maintain IV patency.
    c. Maintain IV heparin.
    d. Monitor for chest pain.

PERSONALIZE IT!!

❖ CHF patients have frequent hospitalizations, accounting for a disproportionate percentage of admissions and health care dollars. CHF is a manageable condition if the patient has the proper education. Examine your unit's patient education information on CHF. Is it user-friendly and thorough? How important is the nursing responsibility of prevention to you?

❖ Imagine you are 37 years old and have just survived an acute MI. Your father died from AMI at age 41. Aside from all the high-tech medical treatment, what are your greatest needs? How will these affect different areas of your life?

CROSSWORD PUZZLE

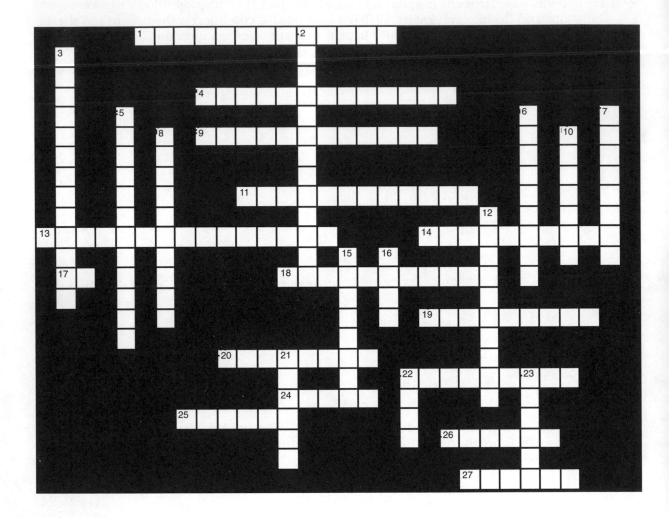

Across

1. Drug used to treat angina.
4. Most common organism causing endocarditis.
9. Heart's ability to beat regardless of external stimuli.
11. Inflammation of the pericardium.
13. Process of fatty plaque accumulating arterial vessels.
14. Type of angina caused by coronary artery spasm.
17. Abbreviation for elevated cardiac enzyme 2–6 hours post-MI.
18. Term for potassium level < 3.5 mEq/L.
19. _____ valve is between the right atrium and ventricle.
20. _____ valve is between the right ventricle and pulmonary artery.
22. _____ edema results from CHF; fluid infiltrates the lungs.
24. Maximum tablet dose of nitroglycerin in a 15-minute period.
25. Sound auscultated when turbulent blood flow through valves.
26. _____ valve is between the left ventricle and aorta.
27. Type of pacemaker that stimulates the heart as needed.

Down

2. Ability of the heart muscle to shorten when stimulated.
3. Classification of drugs given to lyse clots.
5. Inflammation of the inner-most layer of heart muscle.
6. The _____ nervous system exerts control over the cardiovascular system.
7. Angina that worsens over time and often requires intervention.
8. _____ heart failure is indicated by the presence of S_3.
10. Average heart rate is _____ beats per minute.
12. Death of myocardial tissue.
15. Drug given for pain related to MI.
16. Surgical revascularization procedure performed on patients with coronary artery.
21. Valve between the left atrium and ventricle.
22. Interventional procedure that compresses plaque to increase myocardial blood.
23. Chest pain from ischemic heart muscle.

CONCEPT MAP

Complete a comprehensive data map for Mrs. H., a 72-year-old, who was just admitted with increasing dyspnea and confusion. Mrs. H.'s skin is pale and diaphoretic. She has crackles in all lung fields and 4+ pitting edema bilateral lower extremities with clear yellow fluid leakage.

Client Medical Diagnosis

Laboratory Studies

Pertinent History

Predisposing Factors of the Diagnosis

Diagnostic Studies

Prioritized Problem List

Supportive Measures

Definitive Treatment
(possible prescribed meds, treatments, IV fluids)

Chapter 10

NERVOUS SYSTEM ALTERATIONS

LEARNING OUTCOMES

- Review the anatomy and physiology of the central nervous system.
- Describe the pathophysiology and nursing and medical management of patients with increased intracranial pressure.
- Complete an assessment of a critically ill patient with a nervous system injury.
- Describe the pathophysiology and nursing and medical management of patients with head injury.
- Define current nursing and medical therapy for spinal cord injury.
- Discuss the nursing assessment and care of a critically ill patient with cerebrovascular disease.
- Describe the pathophysiology and expected treatment for status epilepticus.

TERMINOLOGY

- anisocoria
- autonomic dysreflexia
- Babinski reflex
- cerebral perfusion pressure (CPP)
- Cheyne-Stokes respirations
- contralateral
- cytotoxic edema
- decerebrate
- decorticate
- dermatome
- Glasgow Coma Scale (GCS)
- hematoma
- herniation syndromes

- hypercapnia (hypercarbia)
- hypocapnia
- ictal/postictal
- infratentorial
- intracranial compliance
- intracranial pressure (ICP)
- ipsilateral
- limbic system
- neuroglia
- plexus
- supratentorial
- vasogenic edema
- Wernicke-Korsakoff syndrome

KEY POINTS

❖ Anatomy and Physiology of the Nervous System

- The neuron is the basic transmitter; three-quarters of the 12 million neurons are located in the cerebral cortex.

- Neuroglial cells are 10 times as numerous as neurons; they form supporting tissues and structures, making up half of the brain and spinal cord.

  - Control ion concentrations

  - Transport nutrients, gases, and wastes

  - Four types: microglia, astrocytes, oligodendrites, and ependymal cells

- Neural cells depolarize and repolarize in similar fashion to cardiac cells; resting membrane potential (RMP) ranges from –60 to –70 millivolts (mV).

- Synapse: the point of junction between neurons where an impulse is transmitted.

  - Three structures are necessary for transmission: Presynaptic terminals, synaptic cleft, and postsynaptic membrane

  - Released neurotransmitters cause excitation, inhibition, or modification of neural response. Common ones are acetylcholine, dopamine, norepinephrine, serotonin, glutamate, and endorphins

- Metabolism: The brain (encephalon) requires a constant O_2 supply; it cannot store O_2. Hypoxia may be reversible, but an anoxic state lasting more than 4 minutes causes permanent damage.

  - Hypercapnia causes dilation of cerebral arteries, resulting in increased intracranial pressure (ICP).

  - Glucose is the brain's main energy source; confusion develops when glucose level drops below 70 mg/100 ml; coma occurs at a level less than 20 mg/100 ml.

- The choroid plexus is highly vascular tissue found in the ventricles of the brain; it forms cerebrospinal fluid (CSF) at a rate of approximately 500 ml/day.

  - About 125 to 150 ml of CSF are typically present in the ventricles and subarachnoid space

❖ Structure and Function

- The scalp is the outermost protective layer; the skull is the rigid cavity that holds the brain (frontal, parietal, temporal, occipital bones).

  - 3 tissue layers or meninges cover the brain: dura mater is the outer and toughest; arachnoid mater is the "spider web" middle layer; pia mater is the inner layer.

  - Epidural and subdural are potential spaces; the subarachnoid space is a real space between the arachnoid and pia mater.

  - The tentorium cerebelli is an extension of the dura mater between the cerebrum and cerebellum that supports the occipital lobes.

- The cerebral hemispheres:

  - Frontal lobes—conscious thought, abstract thinking, judgment, initiation of motor activity

  - Temporal lobes—auditory processing, auditory association (Wernicke's area)

  - Parietal lobes—sensory function, perception, association, and processing

  - Occipital lobes—visual reception and association

  - Basal ganglia—motor control of fine body movement

- Diencephalon: uppermost portion of the brain stem

  - Thalamus—relay station for sensations, except smell

  - Hypothalamus—temperature, water, and hormone regulation; appetite; thirst

- Midbrain: lies between the diencephalon and pons; CN III (occulomotor) and IV (trochlear); reticular activating system (RAS); controls wakefulness.

- Pons: lies between midbrain and medulla oblongata; CN V (trigeminal), VI (abducens), VII (facial), and VIII (vestibulocochlear); controls rate and length of respirations.

- Medulla oblongata: lies between pons and spinal cord; CN IX (glossopharangeal), X (vagus), XI (accessory), and XII (hypoglossal); regulates respiratory rhythm, pulse rate and strength, and vasomotor activity.

- Cerebellum: lies in posterior fossa of the skull; regulates equilibrium, fine movement, muscle tone, and coordination.

- Spinal cord: continuous with medulla oblongata; spinal canal is an extension of the fourth ventricle and contains CSF.

  - 31 segments, each with a pair of spinal nerves

  - Dorsal (posterior) roots = afferent impulse conduction

  - Ventral (anterior) roots = efferent impulse conduction

- Peripheral nervous system (PNS): the portion outside of the CNS

  - 12 pairs of cranial nerves, 31 pairs of spinal nerves, and branches to the entire body

- Autonomic nervous system (ANS):

  - Sympathetic (SNS) thoracolumbar system ("fight or flight"); norepinephrine is main neurotransmitter.

  - Parasympathetic (PNS) system (craniosacral system); dominates nonstress situations; acetylcholine is main neurotransmitter.

❖ Increased Intracranial Pressure (ICP)

- The cranium contains three uncompressible contents: brain tissue, blood, and CSF. Increase in volume of any of these can cause increased ICP (16 mm Hg or greater).

  - Intracranial compliance is a measure of the brain's compensatory mechanisms: increasing CSF absorption, shifting blood to the subarachnoid space, or inhibiting CSF production (chemical and pressure autoregulation).

- Cerebral blood flow (CBF) brings O_2 and glucose to the brain. Decreased CBF can cause ischemia.
  - Cerebral perfusion pressure (CPP) reflects CBF; 60–100 mm Hg range. CPP = mean arterial pressure (MAP) – ICP.
- Cerebral edema is an increase in water content of brain tissue.
  - Cytotoxic edema—intracellular swelling of neurons due to hypoxia and hypoosmolality; failure of sodium-potassium pump (common in DKA).
  - Vasogenic edema—due to breakdown of the blood-brain barrier and increased extracellular fluid space (head injuries, brain tumors, abscesses).
- Herniation is a shifting of the brain from its usual compartment as a result of ICP.
  - Supratentorial herniation:
    - Cingulate—unilateral lesion forces cerebral tissue under falx cerebri to other hemisphere; changes in LOC and mental status.
    - Central—downward shift of hemispheres, basal ganglia, and diencephalon through the tentorial notch; changes in LOC and mental status; increased muscle tone; motor weakness; changes in respiratory pattern; bilateral Babinski reflexes; later, decorticate posture and Cheyne-Stokes respirations.
    - Uncal—unilateral supratentorial lesion forces uncus of temporal lobe through the tentorial notch; unilateral pupil dilation, ipsilateral third nerve palsy, contralateral hemiplegia; later, unresponsive and coma state.
  - Infratentorial herniation:
    - Cerebellar tonsils are displaced through the foramen magnum; fatal damage to respiratory and cardiac centers.
- Nursing assessment:
  - Past history from patient or family of symptoms, onset, progression, and chronology. Medications, past surgeries, environmental exposures and lifestyle habits are important.
  - Clinical manifestations: changes in LOC, speech patterns, pupillary reaction, facial asymmetry, loss of gag reflex.
    - Glasgow Coma Scale (GCS)—the standard assessment tool for LOC; rates eye opening, verbal response, and motor response to standardized stimuli; range 3–15; score of 7 or less indicates coma.
    - Language skills—expressive aphasia, receptive aphasia, global aphasia
    - Memory—short-term and long-term
    - Cranial nerve (CN) function—helpful mnemonic: *On Old Olympus' Towering Tops, A Finn And German Viewed Some Hops;* see exercise at the end of this chapter for CN review.
    - Motor status, spontaneous movement, muscle strength and tone, coordination.
    - Postures and reflexes:
      - Hemiplegia—one side of body stops spontaneous movement; indicates cortical lesion.

- Decorticate rigidity—flexion of upper extremities, extension with internal rotation of lower extremities; indicates cortical, subcortical, or diencephalon lesion.

- Decerebrate rigidity—clenched jaws, full extension of extremities, plantar extension, pronated forearms, wrist and finger flexion; indicates midbrain or pons lesion.

- Bilateral flaccidity—no response.

- Babinski's reflex—major pathological deep tendon reflex; upper motor neuron lesion and damage to the corticospinal tract.

- Vital signs (VS): The patient may suffer severe irreversible damage by the time VS changes are detected.

- ICP monitoring: Benefits must outweigh risks.

  - Intraparenchymal fiberoptic probe—easy insertion and lower incidence of infection, but expensive and fragile.

  - Intraventricular catheter—accurate CSF pressure readings, therapeutic and diagnostic drainage of CSF, but high risk for infection and CSF loss, difficult to insert, and frequent recalibration required.

  - Epidural probe—between skull and dura mater; low risk of infection, but inaccurate pressure readings at high ICP levels.

  - Subarachnoid bolt—in subarachnoid space; easy insertion and accurate CSF pressures, but frequent irrigation required and high risk for infection.

- Waveform monitoring (viewed as trends—not individual waves):

  - A waves (plateau waves) indicate advanced intracranial hypertension. 50 to 100 mm Hg.

  - B waves warn of potential risk of increased ICP; correspond to respirations. Less than 50 mm Hg.

  - C waves lack clinical significance. 16 to 20 mm Hg.

- Hemodynamic monitoring: Assess cerebral perfusion and fluid management.

- Cerebral oxygenation monitoring: Jugular bulb oxygen saturation (SjO$_2$). Normal value = 65%. Values less than 50% suggest cerebral ischemia.

- Medical assessment: ABGs, continuous O$_2$ saturation, CBC, coagulation profile, electrolytes, BUN, creatinine, urinalysis and osmolality; CT scan, skull x-rays, EEG, CBF, and cerebral arteriography.

- Medical interventions include diuretics, corticosteroids, oxygenation, BP management; surgical removal of a mass or lesion, infarcted area, or hematoma may be required.

- Nursing diagnoses may include risk for altered cerebral tissue perfusion; ineffective breathing pattern or impaired gas exchange; ineffective airway clearance; decreased adaptive capacity; altered nutrition, fluid volume deficit; risk for infection; altered thought processes; risk for injury; and ineffective family coping.

- Nursing interventions include maintaining adequate CBF, fluid and electrolyte balance, and ICP within normal range; minimizing hypermetabolic state, muscle loss and impairment of thought processes; protecting from injury, infection and hazards of immobility; and promoting family coping.

  - Assurance, proximity, and information needs are ranked highest for family members.

❖ Head Injury

- Open injuries involve tearing of the scalp, penetration of the meninges, or extension of a fracture into the sinuses or middle ear. Closed injuries involve no break in the scalp (acceleration-deceleration is a common closed injury).

- Skull fractures:

  - Linear—most common; observe for extension and intracranial bleeding.

  - Depressed—inward displacement of outer skull table; may be open or closed; surgical repair needed.

  - Basilar—at the base of the skull, often presents with "raccoon's eyes," Battle's sign, and CSF leaks from nose or ears; dural tears can lead to meningitis.

❖ Brain Injury

- Primary brain injury is the direct result of an impact.

  - Coup injury is the area under direct impact.

  - Contrecoup injury is due to movement of the brain inside the skull—stretching, shearing, rotational tearing forces.

  - Concussion, contusion, diffuse axonal injury, penetrating injury are all primary brain injuries.

  - Hematomas:

    - Epidural—between skull and dura.

    - Subdural—blood collects in subdural space; often a result of a fall in the elderly.

      - Acute subdural—within 48 hours of the injury.

      - Chronic subdural—2 weeks to several months after a low impact injury.

    - Intracerebral—large hemorrhage into brain tissue.

- Secondary brain injury refers to complications resulting from hypoxia, hypotension, anemia, hypercapnia, uncontrolled increased ICP, cerebral edema, hypermetabolic state, infection, or electrolyte imbalance.

- Assessment, diagnosis, and interventions are the same as for increased ICP.

❖ Spinal Cord Injury (SCI)

- Predominantly in males under age 40; result of motor vehicle accidents, sports injuries, falls, gunshot wounds, and diving accidents.

- Causes altered autonomic function, leading to cardiovascular instability (bradycardia, hypotension, venous stasis, loss of temperature control). This is called spinal shock—a temporary loss of autonomic, sensory, and motor function below the level of the lesion.

- An inflammatory reaction leads to cord edema, which compresses spinal cord tissue and vessels. It can ascend or descend from the injury level.

- Complete lesion is total permanent loss below the level of injury.

- Incomplete lesion spares motor and sensory function below the level of injury.

- The higher the level of injury, the greater the functional impairment.

  - Complete lesion at C1–C3 results in ventilator dependency.

  - Complete lesion at C4–C5 causes phrenic nerve damage.

  - Complete lesion below C5 results in intact diaphragmatic breathing.

  - Complete lesion from T1–L2 results in varying amounts of intercostal and abdominal muscle loss.

- Assessment:

  - Assessment of airway, respiratory, and circulatory status is first priority.

  - Next is a neurological assessment of motor ability, reflexes (deep and superficial), and sensory status.

  - Continuous hemodynamic monitoring is needed in the acute period. Body temperature control must also be monitored.

  - GI tract—look for abdominal distention, paralytic ileus, stress ulcers.

  - Bowel and bladder atony occur, as well as urinary retention. Foley catheterization is a usual intervention.

  - Autonomic dysreflexia occurs after spinal shock has ceased in lesions at T6 level or above; it is an exaggerated SNS response to a variety of stimuli. Severe headache, uncontrolled hypertension, and diaphoresis above the level of injury are common symptoms.

- Nursing interventions focus on spinal stabilization, maintaining airway and respiration, and preventing complications of immobility.

❖ Cerebrovascular Disease

- Stroke or cerebrovascular accident (CVA) is the leading cause of brain damage in adults. Treated like a "brain attack."

- Occlusive (ischemic): atherosclerosis results in blockage by thrombus or embolus; early (within 3 hours of onset) administration of thrombolytics improves outcomes.

- Hemorrhagic: ruptured cerebral aneurysm is the most common cause, frequently in the circle of Willis. Chronic HTN is also a cause.

- Arterial-venous malformation (AVM) refers to a congenital defect of abnormal communication between arterial and venous systems without intervening capillaries. AVM is a leading cause of subarachnoid hemorrhage (SAH) and ventricular hemorrhage in young people.

❖ Status Epilepticus and Seizures

- A seizure is an abnormal electrical discharge in the brain caused by CNS irritability.

- Status epilepticus is a life-threatening situation that results when a series of seizures lasting more than 30 minutes occurs, with failure to return to consciousness between attacks. Tonic-clonic seizures are continuous.

  - Most frequently caused by irregular dosing of anticonvulsant medication, from withdrawal from alcohol or sedatives, electrolyte imbalance, azotemia, head trauma, or brain tumor.

  - Initial sympathetic response of epinephrine and norepinephrine can cause cardiac dysrhythmias. Further autonomic dysfunction leads to dehydration and electrolyte loss and depletes energy stores.

    - Neuronal necrosis occurs in prolonged seizures.

    - Renal failure results from rhabdomyolysis and acute myoglobinuria.

    - Hyperkalemia results from increased muscle activity.

- Nursing assessment:

  - Assess neurological, respiratory, and cardiovascular systems.

  - Document length and pattern of seizure; monitor lungs for onset of pulmonary edema; cardiac monitoring; have O_2 and suctioning equipment available.

  - High risk for injury: pad side rails, and keep rails up; do not insert tongue blade between clenched teeth.

- Medical interventions:

  - Monitor EEG, serum electrolytes, serum drug levels, cardiac enzymes, ABGs.

  - Diazepam or lorazepam (longer duration of action) for tonic-clonic seizures; phenytoin (mix only with normal saline); phenobarbitol (respiratory depression—don't use with diazepam); general anesthesia and mechanical ventilation may be needed.

REVIEW QUESTIONS

True/False

1. T F Other than the cerebellum, the CNS structure that regulates motor activity and influences tone and reflexes is the thalamus.

2. T F Hypercapnia and hypoxia cause dilation of cerebral arteries and increase the blood circulation into the brain regardless of actual needs.

3. T F Confusion begins to develop when blood glucose levels drop below 20 mg per 100 ml.

4. T F The hypothalamus controls the rate and length of respirations.

5. T F The brachial plexus comprises spinal nerves C4 to C8 and T1, and innervates the muscles of the neck and shoulders.

6. T F A CPP of 60 mm Hg or lower is considered not only low but also life-threatening.

7. T F The herniation syndrome in which the posterior fossa structures are forced through the foramen magnum is called uncal herniation.

8. T F The most common type of stroke is due to vascular occlusion, whereas hemorrhagic causes account for only 25%.

9. T F Thrombolytic agents may be administered during the first hours after a thrombotic occlusive stroke to prevent damage to neural cells.

10. T F Status epilepticus is often a result of withdrawal from alcohol, sedatives, or anti-convulsant medication.

Multiple Choice

1. Under normal circumstances the cerebral vasculature exhibits pressure and chemical autoregulation. What happens when autoregulation is lost?

   a. Central venous engorgement occurs.
   b. CBF is not affected.
   c. Hypertension increases CBF.
   d. Shunting of CSF is blocked.

2. The subarachnoid space lies between the:

   a. arachnoid and dura mater.
   b. arachnoid and pia mater.
   c. dural layers.
   d. scalp and arachnoid layer.

3. In an adult patient, extension of the great toe toward the head in response to plantar stimulation indicates:

    a. absence of Babinski's reflex.
    b. a lower motor neuron lesion.
    c. presence of Babinski's reflex.
    d. a normal finding.

4. Your patient's ICP is being monitored. While you are providing hygiene measures, you observe that the ICP reading is 18 mm Hg. Your first response is to:

    a. cease stimulating the patient.
    b. continue with hygiene measures since this is a normal reading.
    c. lower the head of the bed to 10 degrees.
    d. raise the head of the bed to 45 degrees.

5. The most important indicator of neuorologic status is:

    a. LOC.
    b. neuromuscular reflexes.
    c. pupillary constriction.
    d. vital signs.

6. One of the most common risks associated with status epilepticus is:

    a. autonomic dysreflexia.
    b. diabetes mellitus.
    c. head injury.
    d. pneumonia.

7. Herniation syndromes can be a life-threatening situation. Which syndrome causes the supratentorial contents to shift downward and compress vital centers of the brain stem?

    a. Central herniation
    b. Cingulated herniation
    c. Tonsillar herniation
    d. Uncal herniation

8. In a patient with increased ICP, which of the following cranial nerves would be assessed for consensual light response, elevation of the eyelids, and eye movement?

    a. I, IX, and X
    b. III, IV, and VI
    c. II, V, and VII
    d. II, VI, and X

9. Mr. H has a closed head injury, and responds to painful stimuli by hyperextending his head, clenching his jaw, and extending both upper and lower extremities. What is this posturing called?

    a. Babinski
    b. Decerebrate
    c. Decorticate
    d. Hemiparetic

10. Rupture of a cerebral aneurysm is a common cause of cerebral bleeds. These aneurysms typically rupture into the:

    a. brain tissue.
    b. parenchymal.
    c. subarachnoid space.
    d. ventricular system.

11. Vasospasm is a narrowing of arteries adjacent to an aneurysm, resulting in ischemia and infarction of brain tissue if unresolved. You are alert to this potential problem; you know that vasospasm usually occurs _____ days after a cerebral aneurysm rupture.

    a. 1 to 2
    b. 21 to 28
    c. 4 to 14
    d. There is no usual time period.

12. A nursing diagnosis of "potential for ineffective breathing pattern" would be appropriate for a patient with a spinal cord injury at what level?

    a. C3
    b. C8
    c. T2
    d. L4

13. A spinal cord injury at the S2–S4 level will most likely cause difficulty with:

    a. breathing.
    b. general movement.
    c. vision.
    d. voiding.

14. An arterial-venous malformation is best described as:

    a. an abnormal shunting of blood from the venous to arterial system.
    b. an abnormal shunting of blood from the arterial to venous system.
    c. a twisted tumor that displaces brain tissue.
    d. a condition in which the circle of Willis is incomplete.

15. A major complication of status epilepticus is:

    a. alkalosis.
    b. hyperglycemia.
    c. hypothermia.
    d. respiratory distress.

Matching—Cranial Nerves

1. _____ I—Olfactory

2. _____ II—Optic

3. _____ III—Oculomotor

4. _____ IV—Trochlear

5. _____ V—Trigeminal

6. _____ VI—Abducens

7. _____ VII—Facial

8. _____ VIII—Acoustic

9. _____ IX—Glossopharangeal

10. _____ X—Vagus

11. _____ XI—Spinal accessory

12. _____ XII—Hypoglossal

a. Movement of eyes

b. Muscles of facial movement and tension on ear bones, lacrimation, salivation, taste.

c. Vision

d. Smell

e. Swallowing, gag, salivation, posterior taste, visceral sensory

f. Movement of head and shoulders

g. Eye and upper eyelid movement; pupillary constriction and accommodation

h. Eye movement

i. Hearing and equilibrium

j. Sensation around ears and viscera; swallow, cough, and gag; main PNS nerve

k. Tongue movement—swallowing and phonation

l. Sensation for face, nose, mouth; muscles of mastication and eardrum tension

PERSONALIZE IT!!

❖ Patient education is extremely important for patients prone to seizure activity. Strict compliance to medication therapy is essential. Review your facility's patient education handouts. What are the restrictions on driving?

❖ Many states are modifying laws concerning mandatory use of motorcycle helmets, some requiring mandatory organ donation if helmets are not worn. What are the implications of such legislation? How do you personally feel about such rulings?

CROSSWORD PUZZLE

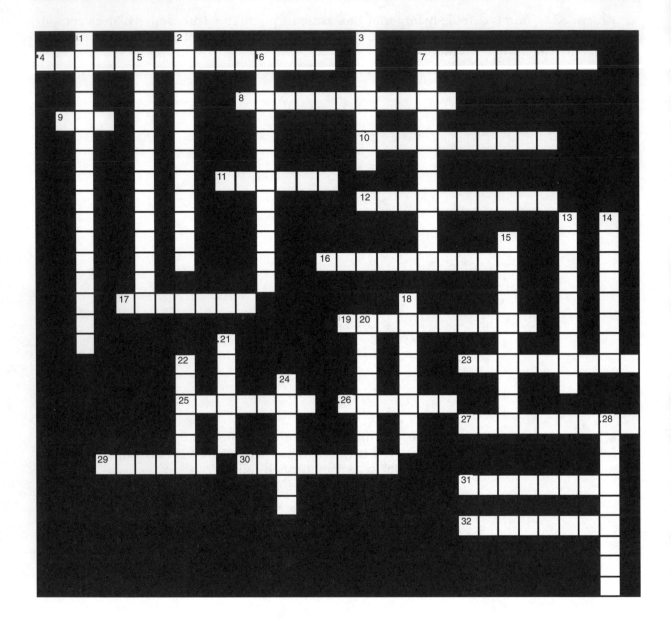

Across

4. Method for draining cerebrospinal fluid with an ICP monitor.

7. Skull fracture in which bone fragments may penetrate the brain.

8. Lay term for stroke (2 words).

9. Reflex that is assessed by asking the patient to say, "Ahh."

10. _____ aphasia is characterized by the inability to talk.

11. _____ aphasia is characterized by the inability to speak or follow directions.

12. Transient loss of consciousness.

16. Diuretic given to reduce ICP.

17. The _____ Coma Scale is a neurological assessment tool.

19. Condition in which lower extremities are paralyzed.

23. _____ dysreflexia is an exaggerated SNS response resulting from injury above T6.

25. A downward shift of the cerebral hemispheres occurs in _____ brain herniation.

26. _____ epilepticus is present when a seizure lasts more than 30 minutes.

27. Brain tissue shifts from one hemisphere to the other in _____ brain herniation.

29. Assessment of reaction to light in the _____ tests the oculomotor nerve.

30. Reflex checked to assess for brainstem function (2 words).

31. Classification of drugs that may be used to treat cerebral edema.

32. Collection of blood between the skull and dura results in this type of hematoma.

Down

1. Most accurate type of ICP monitor.

2. Bolt used to measure ICP.

3. _____ space is the upper limit of normal ICP (mmHg).

5. Hemorrhage into brain tissue.

6. Classification of drugs administered in acute occlusive stroke.

7. Abnormal positioning with legs extended and arms flexed.

13. Bruising of brain tissue.

14. Major pathological deep tendon reflex.

15. Shifting of brain from high to low pressure.

18. Drug used to reduce ICP by withdrawing fluid from normal brain tissue.

20. Nerve controlling hearing and equilibrium.

21. Accessory nerve responsible for movement of the shoulders.

22. Nerve that controls the facial muscles.

24. Skull fracture that occurs at the base of the cranial vault; assessed by clinical symptoms.

28. Cerebral tonsils displace through the foramen magnum in _____ brain herniation.

CONCEPT MAP

Thomas R., a 47-year-old construction worker, was hospitalized after he fell from second-story scaffolding onto a stack of lumber. He has just been admitted to your unit. Initial x-rays show a T2 incomplete spinal cord injury. No head injury is evident from initial diagnostic studies.

Initial Assessment

Baseline Laboratory Tests

Hourly Neurological Assessment

Diagnostic Studies

Possible Complications

Expected Medical Interventions

Pathophysiology of SCI

Autonomic NS response

Biochemical changes

Vascular changes

Nursing Diagnoses

Chapter 11

ACUTE RESPIRATORY FAILURE

LEARNING OUTCOMES

- Describe the pathophysiology of acute respiratory failure.
- Examine the etiology, pathophysiology, assessment, nursing diagnoses, interventions, and outcomes for acute respiratory failure in the patient with:
  - Acute respiratory distress syndrome
  - Chronic obstructive pulmonary disease
  - Asthma
  - Pneumonia
  - Pulmonary embolus
- Formulate a plan of care for the patient with acute respiratory failure.

TERMINOLOGY

- acute respiratory distress syndrome (ARDS)
- alveolar ventilation
- asthma
- atelectasis
- chronic obstructive pulmonary disease (COPD)
- dead space
- deep vein thrombosis
- diffusion defect
- dyspnea
- emphysema
- hemoptysis
- intrapulmonary shunting
- minute ventilation
- neuromuscular blocking agent
- physiological shunt
- pneumoconstriction
- pulmonary toilet
- pulmonary embolism (PE)
- surfactant
- ventilation-perfusion mismatching
- ventilator-associated pneumonia (VAP)

KEY POINTS

❖ Acute Respiratory Failure (ARF)

- ARF is a state of altered gas exchange resulting in abnormal ABG values: PaO_2 < 60 mm Hg, $PaCO_2$ > 50 mm Hg, and pH < 7.30 when the patient is breathing room air.

    - ARF occurs rapidly; chronic failure develops over time and allows compensatory defenses to be activated.

- ARF can result from either failure of oxygenation or ventilation or a combination of both.

    - Failure of oxygenation has several causes:

        - Hypoventilation—leads to reduced alveolar ventilation (drug overdose, neurological disorders, post-surgical pain).

        - Intrapulmonary shunting—return of unoxygenated blood to the left heart when inadequately ventilated lung areas are adequately perfused (septal defects, atelectasis, pneumonia, PE)

        - Ventilation-perfusion mismatching—rate of ventilation (V) should equal rate of perfusion (Q); called V/Q ratio; V/Q mismatching is most frequent cause of hypoxemia.

        - Diffusion defects—result in hypercapnia; CO_2 is more diffusible than O_2 when surfactant and fluid imbalances occur.

        - Decreased barometric pressure, low cardiac output, low hemoglobin, and tissue hypoxia leading to anaerobic metabolism also result in failure of oxygenation.

    - Failure of ventilation is detected by values of $PaCO_2$.

        - Hypoventilation causes accumulation of CO_2 in the alveoli. Respiratory acidosis occurs before renal compensation kicks in.

        - V/Q mismatching results from alteration in amount of dead space in relation to entire tidal volume

- Assessment begins with the neurological system (change in LOC), then respiratory, cardiovascular, nutritional, and psychosocial status.

    - Chest x-rays, pulmonary function tests, electrolytes, CBCs, ABGs, and pulse oximetry are typically ordered.

    - Goals are to maintain airway, optimize O_2 delivery, minimize O_2 demand, treat the cause, and prevent complications.

        - Complications include immobility, medication effects, fluid and electrolyte imbalance, and hazards of mechanical ventilation.

    - Nursing diagnoses include ineffective breathing pattern, impaired gas exchange, risk for infection, fluid volume excess, altered nutrition, skin impairment, anxiety, and ineffective family coping.

❖ Acute Respiratory Distress Syndrome (ARDS)

- Former definition of "acute dyspnea, tachypnea, decreased lung compliance, and diffuse alveolar infiltrates on chest x-ray" has been expanded to include condition, causes, and extent of lung injury.

- Lung injury score involves rating of amount of infiltrates, degree of hypoxemia, amount of positive end-expiratory pressure (PEEP), and static lung compliance.

- ARDS is the most severe degree of lung injury.

- Mortality rate for ARDS is 43% to 70%.

- Causes include sepsis, severe pancreatitis, multiple transfusions, aspiration of gastric contents, abdominal trauma, and multiple fractures. The key clinical finding is respiratory distress that follows a lung insult and is unresponsive to O_2 therapy.

- Pathophysiology of acute and diffuse lung injury:

  - Initial systemic inflammatory reaction occurs. Damage to alveolar-capillary membrane leads to noncardiogenic edema (pulmonary edema), resulting in a stiff, noncompliant lung. Surfactant production decreases due to atelectasis, causing hyperventilation and resultant increase in pulmonary secretions.

  - All of these lead to increased shunting of unoxygenated blood, resulting in tissue hypoxia.

- Early signs of ARDS include restlessness and change in LOC, dyspnea, hyperventilation, cough, and respiratory alkalosis.

- Later, dyspnea becomes severe. Metabolic acidosis results from lactic acid buildup; bilateral patchy infiltrates show on x-ray ("white-out").

- Interventions for ARDS usually include intubation and mechanical ventilation.

  - Lowest possible fraction of inspired O_2 is used.

  - Small tidal volumes are used to prevent barotrauma.

  - Comfort measures may include IV anxiolytic medication and a neuromuscular blocking agent.

  - Close monitoring of fluid and electrolyte balance.

  - Enteral nutrition helps meet increased caloric demands (1.5 to 2.0 times normal).

  - Reassurance and providing information to patient and family are essential.

❖ Chronic Obstructive Pulmonary Disease (COPD)

- COPD is a progressive disease characterized by airflow obstruction, resulting from emphysema or chronic bronchitis. It is the fourth leading cause of death in the United States; its primary cause is cigarette smoke.

- Physiological changes:

  - Permanent enlargement of air spaces

  - Enlargement and increased number of mucus-secreting glands with inflammation and hypertrophy of the mucosal layer of the bronchial tree.

  - Bronchospasm

  - Chronic hypercapnia

  - Right-sided heart failure (cor pulmonale)

- ARF commonly occurs when an exacerbation of COPD is brought on by stressors such as infection, surgery, cardiac disease, or shock.

- Assessment:

  - Look for increased anteroposterior chest diameter (barrel chest), use of accessory muscles for breathing, clubbing of fingertips, diminished lung sounds, wheezes and crackles. Total lung capacity is increased with residual air trapping. X-ray shows low, flat diaphragm.

  - It is important to know baseline ABG levels for a COPD patient when assessing for ARF.

- Interventions include delivery of low concentration O_2 (to avoid blunting the hypoxic drive); beta$_2$-agonists to reverse bronchoconstriction; theophylline; antibiotics for infection; and sedatives to reduce anxiety. Frequent repositioning according to patient tolerance and adequate hydration are important.

- COPD is progressively debilitating, thus continually lowering quality of life. It is important to discuss advance directives and other end-of-life issues with patient and family, hopefully before a crisis arises.

❖ Asthma

- Asthma is a chronic inflammatory disorder of the airways that causes hyperresponsiveness to allergens, viruses, or other irritants.

- Responses are bronchoconstriction, airway edema, mucus plugging, and airway remodeling.

- Results are air trapping, prolonged exhalation, and increased intrapulmonary shunting and V/Q mismatching.

- Asthma is the third leading cause of preventable hospitalizations in the US.

- Assessment

  - Early symptoms include wheezing, dyspnea, cough, and chest tightness.

  - Difficult exhalation causes overinflation of the lungs, which increases dyspnea.

- Interventions

  - Mild exacerbations can be managed with use of short-acting beta$_2$-agonist inhalers.

  - Moderate to severe exacerbations require O_2 therapy, systemic steroids, and bronchodilator inhalers.

  - Status asthmaticus is bronchoconstriction that is unresponsive to bronchodilator therapy and results in ARF.

- Patient education should include monitoring of symptoms, removal of known allergens from the home environment, proper use of inhaler with a spacer, and self-monitoring with a hand-held peak flow meter.

❖ Ventilator-Associated Pneumonia (VAP)

- Nosocomial (hospital-acquired) pneumonia occurs more than 48 hours after admission; its incidence increases drastically in mechanically ventilated patients. This condition is referred to as VAP.

- VAP typically occurs from aspiration of bacteria that colonize the oropharynx and GI tract.

- Diagnosis relies on physical assessment (crackles, dullness in lung fields) and radiographic changes or new onset of purulent sputum.

- The best intervention is prevention. Handwashing remains the most effective preventive method.

- Saline is no longer instilled in the ET tube before suctioning, since this has been found to facilitate entry of bacteria from the ET tube into the respiratory tract.

- Prevention includes maintaining aseptic technique during suctioning, minimizing vent tubing manipulation, and periodically draining tubing condensation away from the patient.

- Reducing aspiration of gastric secretions also helps prevent VAP. Enteral feedings may be dyed to facilitate detection in tracheal secretions. Glucose oxidase reagent strips are also used to detect formula in tracheal secretions.

- Organism-specific antibiotic treatment is necessary for VAP.

❖ Pulmonary Embolism (PE)

- PE is a clot or plug of material that lodges in the pulmonary vasculature. PE may be from a deep vein thrombosis (DVT), a fat embolism from a long bone fracture, septic vegetation, or an iatrogenic catheter fragment.

- PE is classified as massive, submassive, or minor. A massive PE obstructs 50% or more of pulmonary vasculature and usually results in ARF and/or cardiac arrest.

- Virchow's triad refers to three mechanisms that favor development of venous thrombi: venous stasis, hypercoagulability, and vessel wall damage.

- Alveoli beyond the lodging site of a PE lose perfusion but not ventilation (V/Q mismatch); hypoxia damages type II pneumocytes and leads to decreased surfactant production; atelectasis and shunting may follow.

  - Prognosis depends on presence of underlying cardiovascular problems and on the extent of occlusion caused by the PE.

- Assessment: The most common symptoms are chest pain that intensifies upon inspiration; a sudden onset of dyspnea; tachypnea, cough, crackles, hemoptysis; and a sense of impending doom.

- Nursing diagnoses include impaired gas exchange, ineffective breathing pattern, ineffective airway clearance, and anxiety.

- Diagnostics include ABGs, ECG, chest x-ray (pleural effusion is common), V/Q scan, and pulmonary angiography (invasive).

- Treatment:

  - The best therapy is prevention. This includes early postoperative ambulation, pneumatic boots, elastic stockings, checking for Homan's sign (calf pain upon dorsiflexion), and observation for atrial dysrhythmias.

  - Patients at high risk for PE are treated prophylactically with heparin and/or thrombolytic agents.

    - Heparin does not dissolve an existing clot, but prevents enlargement and formation of new thrombi.

- Heparin therapy must be monitored closely with measurement of PTT (partial thromboplastin time).

- If PE occurs, basic ABCs apply (airway, breathing, circulation). Keeping a patent airway and O_2 supplementation are priorities; sometimes surgical intervention is needed.

REVIEW QUESTIONS

True/False

1. T F   V/Q mismatching is the most common cause of hypoxemia in respiratory failure.

2. T F $PaCO_2$ decreases by approximately 4 mm Hg every decade of life.

3. T F   Positioning the patient with unilateral lung disease with the good lung down maximizes perfusion to that side.

4. T F   Changes in personality and disorientation are late changes in patients with ARDS.

5. T F   Tidal volumes larger than 10 ml/kg on mechanical ventilator are recommended for patients with decreased lung compliance as seen in ARDS.

6. T F   Studies have shown that the prone position can improve oxygenation in ARDS patients.

7. T F   Caloric needs of ARDS patients are approximately half the normal values.

8. T F   Bronchospasm and cor pulmonale are frequently seen in patients with COPD.

9. T F   Increased total lung capacity and functional residual capacity, but decreased expiratory flow, are seen in pulmonary function tests on COPD patients.

10. T F   Ventilator associated pneumonia most often results from aspiration of condensation in the ventilator tubing.

Multiple Choice

1. Mrs. Leoni is hospitalized with respiratory distress due to emphysema. She is being treated with O_2 at a rate of 1.5 L/min because:

   a. her alveoli have been damaged and may rupture with higher doses of O_2.
   b. her alveoli cannot absorb higher levels of O_2 due to the emphysema.
   c. her respiratory center requires low O_2 concentration to stimulate breathing.
   d. this is the maximum O_2 concentration that can be given by nasal cannula.

2. Mr. Leoni is visiting his wife at the hospital. When you comment that he is doing pursed lip breathing, he explains that he has COPD. You know this helps him by:

   a. decreasing the amount of air trapped in his alveoli after expiration.
   b. enabling him to lengthen expiration, thus increasing his CO_2 retention.
   c. helping him to lengthen inspiration and shorten expiration.
   d. increasing his CO_2 concentration, which will stimulate his breathing.

3. You would document presence of atelectasis when you hear:

   a. crackles and rhonchi in lung bases.
   b. decreased or absent breath sounds in some areas.
   c. inspiratory stridor.
   d. expiratory wheezes.

4. Symptoms of early respiratory failure are:

   a. cyanosis and pallor.
   b. dyspnea and nasal flaring.
   c. hypertension and bradycardia.
   d. irritability and restlessness.

5. An intrapulmonary shunt occurs with:

   a. inadequate circulation.
   b. inadequate perfusion.
   c. inadequate secretion.
   d. inadequate ventilation.

6. As diffusion capacity is reduced, _____ is first affected.

   a. $PaCO_2$
   b. PaO_2
   c. pH
   d. N

7. Anatomical dead space is normally what percentage of the inspired volume?

   a. 10%–20%
   b. 25%–30%
   c. 40%–50%
   d. 3%–5%

8. The V/Q mismatch and hypoxemia resulting from intrapulmonary shunting initially cause:

   a. decreased airway resistance.
   b. hypocapnia.
   c. hypoventilation.
   d. increased compliance.

9. Baseline ABGs for a COPD patient might show:

   a. PaO_2 50 and $PaCO_2$ 35.
   b. PaO_2 55 and $PaCO_2$ 55.
   c. PaO_2 70 and $PaCO_2$ 50.
   d. PaO_2 75 and $PaCO_2$ 40.

10. Virchow's triad refers to:

    a. the syndrome of ARDS.
    b. mechanisms that identify tamponade.
    c. the syndrome of CHF.
    d. mechanisms that favor the formation of thrombi.

Symptom Identification

Indicate whether the symptom is an early (E) or late (L) sign of ARDS or whether it is present at both times (E, L).

1. _____   Hyperventilation with normal breath sounds

2. _____   Tachycardia

3. _____   Cyanosis

4. _____   Decreased PaO_2

5. _____   Restlessness

6. _____   Decreased PaO_2 with respiratory alkalosis

7. _____   Severe dyspnea

8. _____   Cough

9. _____   Intercostal and suprasternal retractions

10. _____   Crackles, rhonchi

11. _____   Metabolic acidosis

12. _____   Increased peak inspiratory pressures

13. _____   Normal chest x-ray

14. _____   Increased temperature

15. _____   Hypocapnia and hypoxemia

16. _____   Pallor

17. _____   Dyspnea

18. _____   Chest x-ray with bilateral patchy infiltrates

19. _____   Change in behavior, disorientation

20. _____   Decreased functional residual capacity

PERSONALIZE IT!!

❖ Patient education is a fundamental part of asthma management and prevention of acute exacerbation and hospitalization. Self-monitoring with a peak flow meter to measure peak expiratory flow rate and proper use of metered-dose inhalers are two basic interventions that are poorly performed by most patients. Familiarize yourself with these devices so that you will be able to teach their use effectively.

❖ Incidence of childhood asthma has risen dramatically over the last decade. Do you think there is any connection between this rise and environmental factors such as air pollution, food additives, and lack of exercise among young people?

CROSSWORD PUZZLE

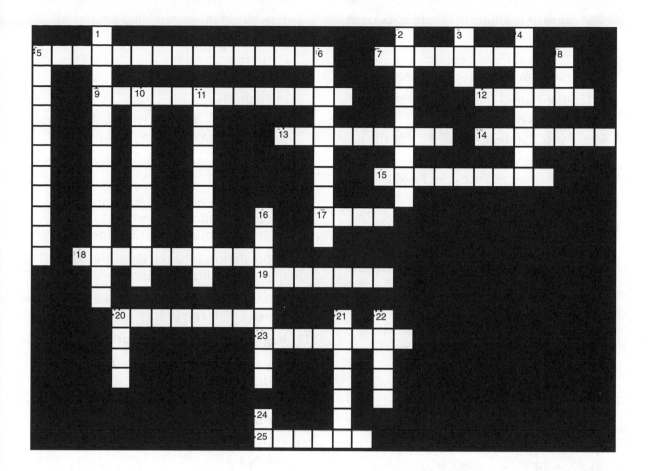

Across

5. The cause of respiratory failure associated with drug overdose.

7. V/Q _____ is the most common cause of hypoxemia in respiratory failure.

9. An initial sign of ARDS is a decreasing level of _____.

12. Chronic inflammatory disorder of the airways.

13. What lung compliance does in ARDS.

14. Primary cause of COPD.

15. The _____ rate for patients diagnosed with ARDS is 43%–70%.

17. Abbreviation for acute respiratory distress syndrome.

18. _____ treatment for VAP should be organism-specific.

19. Clot that travels from larger to smaller vessels.

20. As ARDS progresses, the nurse hears this on auscultation.

23. Noninvasive method of assessing oxygen saturation is pulse _____.

25. Assessment sign associated with DVT.

Down

1. Type of pulmonary edema seen in ARDS.

2. Gas movement from higher to lower concentration.

3. Abbreviation for ventilator-associated pneumonia.

4. Term used to describe the chest x-ray of person with ARDS.

5. Most effective method to prevent VAP in the hospital.

6. Type of pneumonia that occurs > 48 hours after admission to the hospital, excluding prior incubating infections.

8. Abbreviation for exercise of the limbs that may reduce the risk of DVT.

10. System that should be assessed first in the patient with respiratory failure.

11. Respiratory assessment starts with _____.

16. Muscles that patients use in association with COPD or respiratory distress.

20. Abbreviation for disease caused by chronic bronchitis or emphysema.

21. Drug given subcutaneously to reduce the risk of DVT.

22. Positioning used for patients with ARDS to increase perfusion to lungs.

24. Normal value is 7.35–7.45

CONCEPT MAP

Complete a comprehensive data map for Mrs. I, who came to the emergency department by ambulance after her husband found her gasping for breath and in a state of extreme anxiety. She has COPD that is generally under control, but she has had a cold for several days now. Yesterday evening she bruised her shin on a protruding shelf. What findings do you expect to see? What tests do you expect will be ordered?

Client Medical Diagnosis

Laboratory Studies

Pertinent History

Predisposing Factors of the Diagnosis

Diagnostic Studies

Prioritized Problem List

Supportive Measures

Definitive Treatment
(possible prescribed meds, treatments, IV fluids)

Chapter 12

ACUTE RENAL FAILURE

LEARNING OUTCOMES

- Review anatomy and physiology of the renal system.
- Describe the pathophysiology of the three categories of renal failure.
- Identify the systemic manifestations of acute renal failure.
- Describe the physical assessment of the renal system, interpret lab values, and describe radiological diagnostic tests.
- Develop a plan of care for the patient with acute renal failure including nursing management and anticipated outcomes.
- Describe medical management of the patient with acute renal failure.
- Discuss assessment and care of the dialysis patient.

TERMINOLOGY

- acute tubular necrosis (ATN)
- ammonia
- antiemetic
- anuria
- arteriovenous fistula
- arteriovenous shunt
- azotemia
- catabolism
- chemotaxis
- Chvostek's sign
- continuous renal replacement therapy (CRRT)
- creatinine clearance
- dialysate
- disequilibrium syndrome
- dry body weight
- ecchymosis
- erythropoietin
- glomerular filtration
- guaiac
- hematuria
- hemodialysis
- hemofiltration
- intravenous pyelography
- micturition
- nephrosonography
- nocturia
- oliguria
- peritoneal dialysis
- renal osteodystrophy
- uremic encephalopathy
- uremic frost
- uremic halitosis

139

KEY POINTS

❖ Anatomy and Physiology of the Renal System

- The principal organs of the renal system are the kidneys. The nephron is the basic functional unit of the kidney. There are 1 to 3 million nephrons per kidney, each of which is composed of a renal corpuscle (Bowman's capsule and glomerulus) and a tubular structure. 85% of the nephrons are found in the cortex of the kidney; the remaining 15% are found in the medulla and are responsible for the concentration of urine.

- The adrenal glands sit on top of each kidney and produce aldosterone, a hormone which plays a role in sodium and water balance. The kidneys receive 20%–25% of cardiac output or 1200 ml blood/min. The glomerulus is a cluster of minute blood vessels that filter blood. Main processes through which the kidneys maintain homeostasis are:

  - Regulation of fluid and electrolytes and excretion of waste—Blood flows through each glomerulus (where water, electrolytes, and waste products are filtered out), then passes through the glomerular membrane (note: RBCs, albumin, and globulin cannot pass through), into Bowman's capsule and forms glomerular filtrate. Normal glomerular filtration rate (GFR) is 80–125 ml/min. The kidneys produce 180 L of filtrate/day; 99% is reabsorbed. Regulation of electrolyte composition occurs as electrolytes are reabsorbed or secreted. Aldosterone and ADH play a role in water reabsorption. Aldosterone also plays a role in sodium reabsorption. One percent of the original 180 L/day of filtrate is excreted in urine for an average urinary output of 1–2 L/day.

  - Regulation of acid-base balance—Kidneys maintain this balance in three ways: reabsorption of filtered bicarbonate; production of new bicarbonate; and excretion of small amounts of H ions buffered by phosphates and ammonia.

  - Regulation of BP—Special cells known as the juxtaglomerular apparatus, located in the arterioles and distal convoluted tubules, produce renin in response to a decrease in blood flow and sodium ion concentration. Renin activates the renin-angiotensin-aldosterone cascade, which results in angiotensin II production. Vasoconstriction and release of aldosterone occur, raising blood pressure, increasing Na^+ and water reabsorption, and causing excretion of K^+.

❖ Pathophysiology of Three Categories of Acute Renal Failure

- Acute renal failure is a clinical syndrome resulting in a sudden deterioration of renal function with retention of nitrogenous waste (azotemia), accompanied by oliguria (urine output of less than 400 ml/24 hr) Note: 30%–50% of patients with acute renal failure are nonoliguric, but the urine is deficient in solutes and waste. Anuria is urinary output of less than 100 ml/24 hr and is less often seen in acute renal failure. When azotemia (build-up of nitrogenous waste in the blood) progresses to the point where the patient experiences symptoms, the condition is known as uremia.

  - Prerenal acute renal failure results from conditions that interfere with renal perfusion as a result of the following: fluid volume loss, extracellular fluid sequestration (third-spacing), inadequate cardiac output, and vasoconstriction of the renal blood vessels. Common prerenal causes of acute renal failure are (1) volume depletion related to hemorrhage, GI loss, renal loss, volume shifts, (2) vasodilation related to sepsis, anaphylaxis, or drugs; and (3) impaired cardiac performance (CHF, MI, cardiogenic shock, dysrhythmias, pulmonary edema).

- Postrenal acute renal failure results from obstruction of the flow of urine. Increased intratubular pressure results in a decrease in GFR and abnormal nephron function; it usually reverses rapidly once the obstruction is removed. Common causes are BPH, prostate Ca, calculi, etc.

- Intrarenal acute renal failure results when functional kidney tissue is damaged. The most common intrarenal condition is acute tubular necrosis (ATN). It occurs with prolonged ischemia or exposure to nephrotoxic substances (aminoglycocide antibiotics, ACE inhibitors, NSAIDs, etc). Hypoperfusion of the kidney results with severe vasoconstriction and ischemia, damage to the glomerular basement membrane and tubular epithelium, leading to obstruction at the damaged sites. If the ATN is from a nephrotoxic substance, self-repair of the epithelium often occurs.

- Other causes of acute renal failure include glomerulonephritis, vasculitis, and malignant hypertension.

- The pathophysiology of oliguria, which accompanies ATN, consists of five mechanisms: (1) increased renal vasoconstriction; (2) cellular edema; (3) decreased glomerular capillary permeability; (4) intratubular obstruction; and (5) back-leak of glomerular filtrate.

❖ Course of Acute Renal Failure

- Initiation or onset: the time period between the occurrence of the precipitating event until the beginning of change in urine output; lasts several hours to 2 days; damage is potentially reversible.

- Maintenance (oliguric/anuric) phase: intrinsic renal damage has occurred; lasts 8 to 14 days (sometimes much longer); complications of uremia include hyperkalemia and infection; dialysis or CRRT required.

- Recovery (diuretic) phase: renal tissue recovers and repairs itself; lasts 4 to 6 months.

❖ Systemic Manifestations of Acute Renal Failure

- There are two types of clinical presentations depending on underlying causes:

  - Nonoliguria—Patient will present with tachycardia, hypotension, flat neck veins (volume-depleted prerenal cause)

  - Oliguria—Patients present with fluid overload, CHF, pulmonary edema, dysrhythmia, peripheral or systemic edema, and hypertension (intrarenal cause).

- Assessment:

  - Hematological system—anemia, alterations in coagulation, leukocytosis with increased susceptibility to infection, electrolyte imbalances, metabolic acidosis

  - Respiratory system—pneumonia, pulmonary edema

  - GI system—anorexia, nausea and vomiting, stomatitis, uremic halitosis, gastritis, and bleeding

  - Neuromuscular system—drowsiness, confusion (uremic encephalopathy), irritability, coma, tremors, twitching, convulsions

  - Psychosocial system—decreased mentation, concentration, altered perceptions, psychosis

  - Integumentary system—pallor, yellowness, dryness, pruritus, purpura, ecchymosis, uremic frost

- Endocrine system—glucose intolerance

- Musculoskeletal system—hypocalcemia

❖ Methods for Assessing the Renal System

- Physical assessment: Fluid balance—assess body weight, I&O, skin turgor, mucous membranes, breath sounds, edema, JVD.

- Serum and urine lab values (QD): Lab alerts in acute renal failure include hyperkalemia, hyponatremia, hypocalcemia, hypermagnesemia. The best measure of renal function is urinary creatinine clearance (estimated GFR). Normal rate is 80–125 ml/min; a decrease is consistent with renal dysfunction. Analysis of urine sediment and electrolyte levels are helpful in distinguishing between different causes of renal failure. In prerenal there are no cells found, but urine may contain hyaline casts; postrenal urine may contain stones, crystals, sediment, bacteria, and clots. Urine electrolyte levels discriminate prerenal causes and ATN.

- Radiologic tests:

  - Noninvasive—KUB (kidneys, ureters, bladder) reflects size, shape, position, and detects calculi, cysts, tumors. Renal ultrasonagraphy evaluates urinary collecting system for any obstruction.

  - Invasive—IVP, CT, renal angiography, renal scanning, and biopsy

❖ Patient-Centered Care Plan and Anticipated Outcomes

- Diagnoses:

  - Fluid volume excess related to sodium and water retention and excess intake

  - Risk for infection related to depressed immune response secondary to uremia and impaired skin integrity

  - Altered nutrition (less than body requirements) r/t uremia, altered oral mucous membranes, and dietary restrictions

- Two vital nursing interventions include accurate measurement of I&O and daily weights.

- Other important interventions include prevention of infection (occurs in 70% of patients). Do not automatically place indwelling catheters. Do peak and trough levels of drugs to prevent accumulation and toxicity.

- Expected outcomes with appropriate interventions: stable fluid, hemodynamic status, and vital signs; body weight within two pounds of dry weight; normal skin turgor and oral mucosa; serum labs and ABGs WNL; absence of infection; nutritional intake adequate for desired weight.

❖ Medical Management

- Prerenal causes: Prompt treatment of hypovolemia with replacement of fluid, depending on the cause of the loss. Aggressive treatment of sepsis and cardiogenic shock.

- Postrenal causes. Usually resolved with insertion of an indwelling bladder catheter (transurethral or suprapubic) or ureteral stent.

- Management of ATN: Common interventions include diuretics (osmotic or loop—e.g., furosemide), and dopamine; dietary management with protein and electrolyte restrictions; dialysis and continuous replacement therapies; epogen may be used for anemia.

- Drug therapy: Water-soluble drugs (vitamins, cimetidine, phenobarbital) should be administered after dialysis. Drugs that are protein- or lipid-bound or metabolized by the liver (phenytoin, lidocaine, vancomycin) are not removed by dialysis and can be given any time. Antihypertensives are withheld for 4–6 hours before dialysis.

- Dietary management: Energy expenditure with acute renal failure is 30%–50% higher because of catabolism; also dialysis contributes to protein catabolism, and loss of amino acids and water-soluble vitamins. Recommended caloric intake of 30–35 kcal/kg ideal body wt/day (containing all essential amino acids), fluid intake equal to the volume of urine output PLUS 600–1000 cc/day.

- Fluids: Salt and water restrictions, diuretics, and low-dose dopamine.

- Electrolyte imbalances:

  - Hyperkalemia—The only two methods effective to reduce plasma K^+ and total body K^+ are dialysis and use of cation exchange resins (Kayexalate).

  - Hyponatremia is treated with fluid restriction.

- Acid-base imbalance—Metabolic acidosis is the primary acid-base imbalance seen in acute renal failure. The goal is to raise the PH to greater than 7.20, in order to avoid the adverse effects of acidosis.

- Dialysis is the primary treatment for acute renal failure. It is defined as the separation of solutes by differential diffusion through a semipermeable membrane placed between two solutions. Types of dialysis:

  - Hemodialysis (most frequently used)

  - Continuous renal replacement therapy (CRRT)

  - Peritoneal dialysis

- Dialysis is initiated early, before uremic complications arise. Access: percutaneous catheters (most common), arteriovenous fistulas, grafts, and shunts. Nursing responsibilities r/t vascular access sites include protection of the site (no blood draws, BPs, IVs, IMs on the extremity where the site is located). With an A-V fistula, the site is auscultated for a bruit, and palpated for thrill every eight hours.

- Complications of hemodialysis include extreme fatigue, hypotension (occurs in 10%–50% of patients), dysrhythmias, muscle cramps, decrease in oxygen content of the blood, infections (vascular access site and hepatitis C), hemolysis, air embolism and hyperthermia.

- Dialysis disequilibrium syndrome might occur after one or two dialysis treatments as a result of the cerebral edema created through an osmotic pressure gradient, which allows fluid to enter the brain until concentrations equal the extracellular fluid. Symptoms include headache, nausea and vomiting, twitching, mental confusion, and occasional seizures.

- CRRT: Continuous ultrafiltration of fluids and clearance of uremic toxins. It is used in ICU when CV status is too unstable for rapid fluid removal. Complications include electrolyte and acid-base imbalances, fluid imbalances, depletion of vitamins, amino acids, hemorrhage, infection, hypothermia, clotting of the filter, rupture or leakage of the filter, and air embolism.

- Peritoneal dialysis: Infusion of dialysate through permanent catheter. Individualized therapy, slower balancing of electrolytes. Convenient for home therapy. Complications: mechanical, metabolic, and inflammatory. Peritonitis is the most frequent complication.

REVIEW QUESTIONS

True-False

1. T F Hypocalcemia is the most life-threatening complication of acute renal failure because it can cause seizures.

2. T F A major goal of nutritional management of acute renal failure is to reduce catabolism of the body's fat sources.

3. T F The best measure of renal function is urinary creatinine clearance.

4. T F Thirty to fifty percent of patients with acute renal failure are nonoliguric and may excrete 2–4 L of normal urine in 24 hours

5. T F Continuous renal replacement therapy (CRRT) is the most frequently used therapy in acute renal failure because it provides continuous ultrafiltration of fluids and clearance of toxins.

6. T F The nursing assessment of a patient with an A-V fistula includes auscultation of the site (for a bruit) and palpation (for the presence of a thrill) every eight hours.

7. T F Peak and trough drug levels are monitored in patients with acute renal failure to avoid suboptimal drug levels since many drugs are removed by dialysis.

8. T F Complications of hemodialysis include hypotension, dysrhythmias, and muscle cramps

9. T F The cause of renal anemia is iron deficiency, for which most patients receive oral iron supplements.

10. T F Patients with acute renal failure who are oliguric have an increased susceptibility to life-threatening infection and therefore should have a catheter inserted immediately using strict aseptic technique.

Multiple Choice

1. Fluid restriction in acute renal failure is determined based on:

   a. daily serum Na levels.
   b. daily weights obtained the same time each day on the same scale.
   c. urine output in a 24-hour period plus insensible losses.
   d. all of the above.

2. The patient's creatinine clearance is 5 ml/min. This data signifies:

   a. normal renal function.
   b. renal dysfunction.
   c. inaccurate lab results.
   d. hyperactive kidneys.

3. Altered nutrition in acute renal failure is related to which of the following?

   a. Energy requirements in catabolic patients 30%–50% higher than basal requirements
   b. GI irritation, stomatitis, and metallic taste in the mouth
   c. Dyspnea and Kussmaul's respiration
   d. Dysphagia due to altered neurological status

4. An elevated BUN may cause body temperature to be:

   a. elevated.
   b. subnormal.
   c. normal.
   d. labile.

5. Acute tubular necrosis (ATN) is potentially reversible in the:

   a. maintenance phase.
   b. recovery phase.
   c. initiation phase.
   d. convalescent phase.

6. Insertion of a ureteral stent would most likely be done for a patient with:

   a. prerenal azotemia.
   b. intrarenal azotemia.
   c. postrenal azotemia.
   d. intrinsic azotemia.

7. Hyponatremia is the result of:

   a. dehydration.
   b. sodium excess.
   c. water overload.
   d. potassium deficit.

8. Signs and symptoms of metabolic acidosis include:

   a. bradycardia, with decreased respiration, low serum bicarbonate, and elevated pH.
   b. Kussmaul's respiration, low pH, and low serum bicarbonate.
   c. lethargy, tachypnea, and elevated serum bicarbonate.
   d. slowed respirations and low pH.

9. Complications of dialysis include all of the following *except*:

   a. dialysis disequilibrium syndrome.
   b. hypertension.
   c. infection.
   d. hemolysis.

Matching—Key Terms

1. _____ Aminoglycoside antibiotics

2. _____ Antihypertensives

3. _____ Metabolic acidosis

4. _____ Acute tubular necrosis

5. _____ Uremia

6. _____ Hyponatremia

7. _____ Azotemia

8. _____ Prerenal

9. _____ Oliguria

10. _____ Hyperkalemia

a. Refers to the presence of nitrogenous waste in the blood.

b. The toxic condition resulting from retention of nitrogenous substances.

c. Urine output of less than 400 ml in 24 hrs.

d. The most common intrarenal condition, resulting from prolonged ischemia.

e. Category of acute renal failure that includes hypovolemia and cardiogenic shock.

f. Exposure to this nephrotoxic substance might result in ATN.

g. Management of this electrolyte imbalance involves use of cation exchange resins.

h. Decreased cardiac contractility results from this imbalance found in acute renal failure.

i. A fluid restricted diet is necessary for patients with acute renal failure related to this electrolyte imbalance.

j. It is recommended that this class of drugs be withheld for 4–6 hours prior to dialysis.

PERSONALIZE IT!!

❖ Your African-American patients are especially prone to having hypertension, which can ultimately lead to acute renal failure if not consistently treated. Few patients are aware of the connection. You can incorporate this into your patient teaching for anyone who has hypertension.

❖ Many ICU patients must undergo dialysis. Ask permission to accompany your patient during the process. Dialysis nurses can share a great deal of specialized knowledge if you are sincerely interested.

CROSSWORD PUZZLE

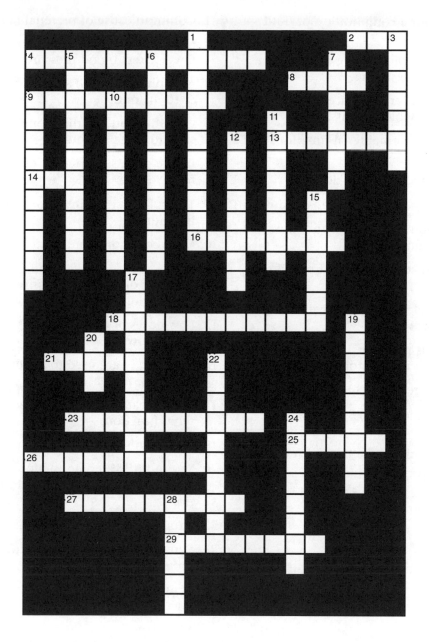

Across

2. Abbreviation for a complication of fluid overload.

4. Most common treatment for renal failure in the critical care setting.

8. Abbreviation for renal replacement therapy used in unstable patients.

9. Phase in which normal renal functions begins to decline.

13. Glands that sit above each kidney.

14. Most common cause of intrarenal failure.

16. Sudden deterioration of renal function causes metabolic _____.

18. Most common complication of peritoneal dialysis.

21. Sound auscultated over arteriovenous graft or fistula.

23. Type of dialysis performed via removal of solutes through the peritoneum.

25. Hormone that regulates blood pressure.

26. Loop diuretic commonly given in renal failure.

27. Type of renal failure resulting from urine obstruction.

29. Volume _____ is common in renal failure and is caused by fluid retention.

Down

1. Common cause of prerenal failure.

3. If a patient has a _____ in his or her arm, never assess blood pressure there.

5. ATN phase with GFR at approximately 5–10 ml/min.

6. Classification of drugs commonly responsible for renal failure.

7. Intake of this nutrient is often limited in renal failure.

9. Type of renal failure caused by damage to the kidney.

10. Most common complication of renal failure.

11. Osmotic diuretic commonly given in renal failure.

12. Low doses of this drug improve renal blood flow.

15. Daily _____ are used to validate intake and output measurements.

17. _____ clearance is the best assessment of renal function.

19. Electrolyte often elevated in renal failure.

20. Serum test of renal function may be falsely elevated in dehydration (abbreviation).

22. Drug given to treat hyperkalemia.

24. Renal failure caused by interference with renal perfusion.

28. Drug given to increase red blood cell production.

CONCEPT MAP

Complete a comprehensive data map for Mrs. D., a 76-year-old white female with a 12-year history of IDDM. Mrs. D. is currently being treated with gentamicin IV x 2 weeks.

Client Medical Diagnosis

Laboratory Studies

Pertinent History

Predisposing Factors of the Diagnosis

Diagnostic Studies

Prioritized Problem List

Supportive Measures

Definitive Treatment
(possible prescribed meds,
 treatments, IV fluids)

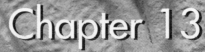

Chapter 13

HEMATOLOGICAL AND IMMUNE DISORDERS

LEARNING OUTCOMES

- Explain the normal anatomy and physiology of the hematological and immune systems.
- Describe pathophysiological changes that affect hematological and immunological structure and function.
- Discuss the risk factors, pathophysiological process, clinical findings, nursing care, and medical management of anemia, neutropenia, malignant white blood cell disorders, human immunodeficiency virus, thrombocytopenia, and disseminated intravascular coagulation.
- Develop plans of care for the immunocompromised host or patient who has a bleeding disorder.

TERMINOLOGY

- acral cyanosis
- active versus passive immunity
- adhesion
- aggregation
- AIDS
- anemia
- chemotaxis
- complement proteins
- cytokine
- disseminated intravascular coagulation (DIC)
- erythropoietin
- fibrinogen

- fibrinolysis
- hematopoiesis
- immunocompromised
- lymphoreticular system
- monokines
- opsonization
- phagocytosis
- reticulocytes
- suppuration
- thrombocytopenia
- thrombopoietin
- tissue anergy

153

KEY POINTS

❖ Hematologic Anatomy and Physiology

- Hematopoiesis is the formation and maturation of blood cells. Formation is mainly in bone marrow, but the spleen, liver, thymus, lymphatic system, and lymphoid tissues are secondary organs.

    - In children, most bones are filled with blood-forming red marrow; in adults, only the vertebrae, skull, chest cage, ilium, and proximal long bones produce blood cells.

    - Hematopoietic stem cells differentiate into erythrocytes, leukocytes, or thrombocytes.

- Blood has four major components: plasma (55% of volume), circulating solutes, serum proteins, and cells (45% of volume).

- Hematopoietic cells:

    - Erythrocytes, or red blood cells (RBCs), are small, biconcave, and anucleate and contain hemoglobin. Their formation is regulated by erythropoietin, which is secreted by the kidneys in response to a perceived decrease in perfusion or tissue hypoxia.

        - Reticulocytes are immature RBCs released early when the demand exceeds the supply of available mature cells.

        - O_2 transport is the main function of RBCs; the affinity of hemoglobin for O_2 depends on blood pH, body temperature, and concentration of 2,3 diphosphoglycerate (2,3-DPG).

    - Platelets (thrombocytes) are the smallest formed elements of the blood. Most circulate freely, but a reserve is stored in the spleen. Platelets are the first responders in the clotting mechanism, forming a platelet plug. They release mediators such as epinephrine and serotonin (vasoconstriction), adenosine diphosphate (platelet adhesion and aggregation), and calcium and phospholipids (clotting).

    - Leukocytes, or white blood cells (WBCs), are larger and less numerous and have nuclei. They have a key role in defense against infective organisms.

        - Granulocytes (polymorphonuclear) leukocytes:

            - Neutrophils—60% to 70% of WBCs. Neutrophils are phagocytic cells that recognize, ingest, and kill microorganisms. Normally there is a majority of segmented neutrophils and fewer band (immature) cells. "Shift to the left" refers to an increased number of band neutrophils, usually indicating an acute bacterial infection.

            - Eosinophils—1% to 5% of WBCs. Eosinophils are active in defense against parasites, and they decrease the severity of allergic reactions. They respond to chemotactic mechanisms (chemical mediators).

            - Basophils—0% to 1% of WBCs. Basophils are important in systemic allergy and inflammatory responses. They contain large granules with heparin, serotonin, and histamine.

- Nongranular leukocytes:

  - Monocytes—1% to 8% of WBCs. Monocytes are the largest nongranular leukocytes. They mature into tissue macrophages (phagocytic scavenger cells). In the lung, they are alveolar macrophages; in the liver, Kupffer's cells; in connective tissue, histiocytes.

  - Lymphocytes—20% to 40% of WBCs. Lymphocytes provide defense against microorganisms, delayed hypersensitivity reactions, autoimmune diseases, and foreign tissue rejection.

    - B lymphocytes mediate humoral immunity; they originate and mature in bone marrow.

    - T lymphocytes mediate cellular immunity; they originate in marrow, mature in the thymus, then reside in lymphoid tissue (long-term immunity).

    - Natural killer cells work in surveillance and destruction of virus-infected and malignant cells.

❖ Immunological Anatomy and Physiology

- Immunity is the body's ability to resist and fight infection. Immune activity requires both WBC response and the lymphoreticular system, which consists of lymphoid tissue, lymphatic channels and nodes, and phagocytic cells.

  - Recognition and destruction of nonself molecules or antigens are the key activities of the immune system. Antigens can be microorganisms, abnormal cells, vaccines, or nonhuman molecules such as penicillin.

    - Autoimmunity: the body sees itself as foreign, as in systemic lupus erythematosus.

    - Active immunity: the body actively produces cells and mediators to destroy the antigen.

    - Passive immunity: transferred from another person (maternal antibodies).

  - Nonspecific defenses are the first line of protection, such as intact skin and mucosal barriers. Second-line defense involves phagocytosis and inflammation. When cellular injury occurs, a process called chemotaxis generates a mediator and a neutrophil response.

    - Mediators include histamine, seratonin, kinins, lysosomal enzymes, prostaglandin, clotting factors, and complement proteins; reactions to mediators cause the redness, heat, and swelling of inflammation.

    - Phagocytes are attracted to the area of injury by the mediators. Opsonization occurs, in which antibody and complement proteins attach to the phagocytic cells to enhance their ability to engulf bacteria.

    - Cytokines are released, including interleukins, tumor necrosis factor, colony-stimulating factors, and interferons. Monocytes and macrophages produce monokines; lymphocytes produce lymphokines.

  - Specific defenses of humoral and cellular immunity take over when nonspecific defenses fail.

- Humoral immunity is mediated by B lymphocytes. Antibodies (immunoglobulins) are formed in response to specific antigens that bind to their receptor sites. There are five classes of immunoglobulins:

  - IgG: most abundant, opsonizes bacteria; crosses placenta.

  - IgM: principle early antibody (7–10 days), causes antigen clumping and activates the complement cascade.

  - IgA: present in seromucous secretions; first antibody formed, but fades as IgG increases.

  - IgE: binds to mast cell surfaces, stimulates histamine release during allergic reactions.

  - IgD: activates B lymphocytes, which produce immunoglubulins.

  - Both primary (memory-stimulating) and secondary (long-term) humoral responses occur.

- Cell-mediated immunity is mediated by the T lymphocyte; it is a delayed reaction. Important in viral, fungal, and intracellular infections and in transplant rejection.

  - T lymphocytes differentiate into helper/inducer T cells, suppressor T cells, and killer cells (which release cytotoxic substances that cause cell lysis).

- Hemostasis is a process involving hematological and nonhematological factors that form a platelet or fibrin clot to control blood loss. Three triggers to the clotting mechanism are tissue injury, vessel injury, and presence of a foreign body in the bloodstream.

  - Vasoconstriction is the initial response; serotonin is released from the vascular wall for a temporary (2–5 hour) clot. Platelets aggregate, releasing adenosine diphosphate (ADP), which stimulates the coagulation proteins to create a fibrin clot.

- Coagulation occurs by intrinsic and extrinsic pathways that share a "final" pathway to clot formation.

  - Intrinsic pathway (initiated by factors from within): Exposure to subendothelial collagen activates factor XII, initiating coagulation.

  - Extrinsic pathway (outside factors): Tissue injury precipitates release of tissue factor, or thromboplastin (factor III) and phospholipids.

  - Both pathways lead to activation of factor X, which converts prothrombin (factor II) to thrombin, then converts fibrinogen (factor I) to fibrin, forming a fibrin mesh and blood clot. Thrombin stimulates platelet aggregation and the activity of other factors and initiates the fibrinolytic system by converting plasminogen to plasmin.

- Procoagulation forces (thrombin is most powerful) must be balanced by anticoagulation factors (fibrin threads that absorb most of thrombin during clot formation and antithrombin III). If plasma protein levels are low, clotting may become inappropriately widespread, as in disseminated intravascular coagulation (DIC).

❖ Hematological and Immunological Systems—Assessment and Interventions

- A complete health history is recorded, noting risk factors such as allergies, anemia, occupational exposure to hazardous substances or radiation, delayed wound healing, liver or renal disease, neoplastic disease, prior surgeries or blood transfusion, and medications.

- Physical examination: general appearance, signs of fatigue, acute illness, or chronic disease. Look for signs of altered oxygenation (dizziness, confusion, lethargy), dyspnea or tachypnea, bleeding or clotting tendencies, altered nutrition (nausea, diarrhea), hematuria, arthritis, and muscle fatigue.

- Diagnostic tests: CBC with differential and coagulation profile are basic screening tests. More invasive examinations (bone marrow) are reserved for cases of inconclusive lab results or suspicion of abnormalities in cellular maturation.

- Nursing priorities include maintaining adequate tissue perfusion, oxygenation, and gas exchange; avoiding infection; providing adequate hydration and skin care; avoiding of transfusion reaction; and treating pain.

❖ Selected Hematologic Disorders

- Anemia is a reduction in numbers of circulating RBCs or hemoglobin that leads to inadequate oxygenation of tissues. Anemia can be mild, moderate, or severe; it can be chronic or acute. Anemia is caused by blood loss, deficient production, abnormal function, or premature lysis. Decreased circulating volume manifests as low central venous pressure and orthostasis and shunting from skin to vital organs

  - Aplastic anemia (stem cell failure)—May be caused by exposure to drugs, chemical, or viruses, or it may be idiopathic. Bruising, nosebleeds, petechiae, and decreased ability to fight infection are common.

  - Hemolytic anemia (increased extrasplenic destruction of or sequestration of RBCs)—Can result from liver or renal disease, hereditary shape disorders, autoimmune disease, drugs, burns, cardiopulmonary bypass, or prosthetic valves. Includes subtype of sickle cell anemia.

  - Pernicious anemia (decreased production of gastric HCL and intrinsic factor; inhibits B_{12} absorption)—Can be hereditary, autoimmune, or post-gastric surgery. Results in weakness, stomatitis, and paresis. Schilling test is specific for pernicious anemia.

  - Folic acid and iron deficiency anemias are related to dietary deficiencies.

- Medical interventions for severe anemias may include blood transfusions, splenectomy, bone marrow transplantation, and synthetic erythropoietin. In the future, intervention may include gene therapy.

❖ White Blood Cell and Immune Disorders

- An immunocompromised patient is one with defined quantitative or qualitative defects in WBCs or immune physiology. Immunodeficiency may be congenital or acquired. Lack of normal inflammatory, phagocytic, antibody, and cytokine responses make infection the leading cause of death in this group. Typical signs such as erythema, swelling, and exudate formation are generally absent or masked.

  - Primary immunodeficiency exists in the immune system.

  - Secondary (acquired) immunodeficiencies result from factors outside the immune system that cause loss of immune function.

- In the critical care environment, an already immunocompromised patient is further challenged by invasive procedures, inadequate nutrition, and exposure to opportunistic pathogens.

- Nursing interventions focus on protecting the patient from infection. Diet should not include raw fruits or vegetables, which might harbor bacteria; plants and flowers also are potential contaminants.

- Invasive lines pose the most common risk for iotrogenic infection; meticulous sterile technique must be maintained.

- Skin integrity and mucous membranes are at risk due to immobility.

- Medical interventions for primary immunodeficiencies involve B cell and T cell replacement therapy or bone marrow transplantation. IgG levels of less than 300 mg/dl warrant immunoglobin infusion. For secondary immunodeficiencies, the underlying cause (such as malnutrition) is treated.

  - Prophylactic antimicrobial agents are administered during periods of high risk for infection.

- Neutropenia is a common finding in immunocompromised patients; it is defined as an absolute neutrophil count less than 1000 cells/mcl of blood. Degrees of neutropenia are mild (500–1000), moderate (100–499), and severe (less than 100).

  - Common causes are overwhelming infections, radiation, exposure to drugs and chemicals, or disease states (aplastic anemia, multiple myeloma, uremia).

  - Symptoms are atypical; fatigue and general malaise accompany dropping counts. Systemic infection presents with hyperthermia, chills, and tachycardia.

  - WBC differential with an absolute neutrophil count is the diagnostic test for suspected neutropenia.

  - Medical treatment for patients receiving antineoplastic or antiretroviral therapy may be given colony-stimulating factors, which enhance bone marrow regeneration of granulocytes. Prophylactic antimicrobials, broad-spectrum agents for known infection, and granulocyte transfusions are also options.

- Malignant WBC disorders:

  - Common risk factors include genetic mutations, viral infection, radiation, carcinogens, benzene derivatives, pesticides, and T lymphocyte immune suppression.

  - Common assessment is an alteration in the immunological response to injury or microbes. Inflammatory response to pathogens is minimal.

  - Oncological emergencies may be a result of the cancer itself, the treatment, or tumor lysis. Anxiety and anticipatory grieving are added to the nursing diagnoses of risk for infection, altered perfusion, and ineffective coping. Few therapies for hematological malignancies are considered curative. Remission is the goal.

  - Malignant WBC disorders include leukemia, lymphoma, multiple myeloma.

    - Leukemia is an overproduction of malignant WBC precursors in the bone marrow. Acute = proliferation of immature cells. Chronic = proliferation of mature cells. Classified according to origin (lymphocytic or nonlymphocytic).

      - All leukemia patients are considered late-stage due to systemic effects. Bone pain is common.

    - Lymphoma affects mature lymphocytes in lymph nodes. Hodgkins can be cured; non-Hodgkins is less curable. Classified by number of lymph nodes involved.

- Multiple myeloma is a disseminated neoplasm of marrow plasma cells (immunoglobulin-producing macrophages). Classified as limited or extensive depending on plasma viscosity, bone manifestations, hypercalcemia, and renal involvement.

    - Bence Jones protein is detected in urine.

- AIDS is a secondary (acquired) deficiency; the HIV retrovirus transcribes its genetic material into host cells, leading to depletion of helper T cells and macrophages essential to the immune response. Decreasing CD_4 cell counts make the patient more susceptible to opportunistic infections, malignancies, and neurological disease.

    - Diagnosis of HIV infection involves detection of core antigen or antibodies to HIV, detected by ELISA and confirmed by Western blot test.

    - CDC criterion for AIDS versus HIV infection is the presence of CD_4 count of less than 200/mcl and the presence of an indicator condition.

    - Medical interventions are primarily antiretroviral medications categorized as nucleoside analogs, nonnucleoside reverse transcriptase inhibitors (NNRTIs), and protease inhibitors. Management of opportunistic infection and monitoring for adverse drug reactions are essential. Average life expectancy is now 11 years.

    - Potential risk of exposure and physical and emotional demands necessitate ongoing psychosocial support for nursing staff.

- Bleeding disorders (coagulopathies) are caused by abnormalities in one of the stages of clotting: vasoconstriction; creation of a platelet plug; development of the fibrin clot; or fibrinolysis. May be inherited (hemophilia, von Willebrand's disease) or acquired (vitamin K deficiency, DIC).

    - Careful medical and social history is taken. Note current medications; history of renal, hepatic, or GI problems; malnutrition.

        - Mucous membranes bleed easily as a result of capillaries lying close to the membrane surface. Look for petechiae.

    - Diagnostics: CBC for quantitative values of RBCs and platelets; PT and PTT; sometimes bleeding time or fibrin degradation products testing will be done.

    - Nursing diagnoses include risk for bleeding, altered protection, fluid volume deficit, pain, decreased tissue perfusion, altered self-image.

    - Medical interventions depend on suspected cause. Component-specific blood replacement is preferred over whole blood (to prevent volume overload and provide more specific treatment).

        - When cause is unknown, local (absorbent gels or topical thrombin) or systemic procoagulant therapies (vasoconstrictors, clot formation enhancers, or breakdown inhibitors) are used.

    - Nursing interventions include maintaining fluid volume and limiting invasive procedures (Foley catheters, rectal temperatures).

    - Thrombocytopenia is a platelet count below 100,000/μL; often asymptomatic above 50,000/μL. May be caused by decreased production in bone marrow, increased destruction, or sequestration in the liver or spleen.

    - Spontaneous bleeding may occur at counts below 20,000–30,000/μL. High risk for fatal hemorrhage occurs at counts below 10,000/μL.

- Platelet transfusion is the key treatment. If multiple transfusions are needed, single-donor products are preferred. Platelet count should increase 10,000–30,000/μL for each unit administered.

- Disseminated intravascular coagulation (DIC) is a serious disorder characterized by exaggerated microvascular coagulation, depletion of clotting factors (thus the name "consumptive coagulopathy"), and subsequent bleeding. When symptoms are acute and severe, mortality rate is 80% to 90%.

  - Common causes of acute DIC are sepsis, multitrauma, and burns.

  - Chronic form is caused by malignancy or renal, liver, or metabolic disease.

  - Subacute form is asymptomatic, found by microscopic examination.

  - Procoagulants are released, activating intrinsic or extrinsic pathways. Large amounts of thrombin are produced, resulting in deposition of fibrin, consumption of clotting factors, and stimulation of fibrinolysis.

  - Clotting in microvasculature causes organ ischemia and necrosis; skin, lungs and kidneys are most often damaged. Thrombophlebitis, PE, CVA, GI bleed, and renal failure may also result.

  - Fibrinolysis releases fibrin degradation products, which are potent anticoagulants that interfere with thrombin, fibrin, and platelet activity. Inability to form clots predisposes the patient to hemorrhage.

  - Diagnosis is based on risk factors, symptoms, and lab results showing prolonged bleeding times, factor depletion and elevated fibrin degradation product (FDPs), increased D-dimer, or decreased antithrombin III.

  - Medical interventions include correction of hypotension, hypoxemia, and acidosis, as well as treatment of infection if it is underlying cause.

    - Blood volume expanders and crystalloid IV fluids (lactated Ringer's or NS) are given to correct hypovolemia.

    - Platelet infusions are a high priority since they provide clotting factors needed for initial platelet plug.

    - Fresh frozen plasma provides fibrinogen (contains all factors and antithrombin III). However, factor VIII may be inactivated by freezing and is provided as cryoprecipitate.

    - Packed RBCs replace cells lost by hemorrhage.

    - Use of heparin in DIC is controversial. Synthetic antithrombin III and aminocaproic acid (Amicar) may be effective in some cases.

  - Nursing interventions include ongoing assessment for thrombotic or hemorrhagic complications. Psychosocial support of family and patient are also crucial, since mortality is high and few survivors of DIC escape functional deficits.

REVIEW QUESTIONS

Multiple Choice

1. In the primary immune response, the principal early antibody seen is:

   a. IgA.
   b. IgD.
   c. IgG.
   d. IgM.

2. Common symptoms for a patient with anemia include:

   a. chest pain, fatigue, orthopnea.
   b. fatigue, dyspnea, tachycardia.
   c. inspiratory pain, hematemesis, tachycardia.
   d. orthopnea, inspiratory pain, pallor.

3. Which nursing diagnosis reflects the stimulus for the body's response of erythropoiesis?

   a. Decreased cardiac output related to myocardial ischemia
   b. High risk for bleeding secondary to anticoagulated state
   c. Impaired tissue perfusion related to hypoxia
   d. Pain related to bone metastasis

4. Folate deficiency anemia can be distinguished from vitamin B_{12} deficiency (pernicious) anemia by the presence of:

   a. Bence Jones protein.
   b. cardiac dysrhythmias.
   c. fatigue.
   d. neurologic impairment.

5. A platelet count of _____/μL would represent a high risk for fatal hemorrhage.

   a. 10,000
   b. 30,000
   c. 50,000
   d. 100,000

6. Humoral immunity is mediated by:

   a. B lymphocytes.
   b. T lymphocytes.
   c. Plasma cells.
   d. Kupffer cells.

7. You are caring for a patient in isolation who has been diagnosed with neutropenia. What signs of infection would you expect to see?

   a. Fever
   b. Heat, redness, and pain
   c. Increased phagocytic activity
   d. Increased WBC levels

8. Mr. Mills is hospitalized with severe urosepsis. In spite of aggressive treatment, he is showing signs of decreased perfusion. Which of the following symptoms would lead you to suspect DIC?

   a. Hypertension, respiratory alkalosis
   b. Increased urinary output, flushed face
   c. Nausea, diarrhea, abdominal cramping
   d. Peripheral cyanosis, oozing from old puncture sites

9. Treatment of secondary immunodeficiencies includes:

   a. B- and T-cell replacement therapy.
   b. bone marrow transplants.
   c. somatic gene therapy.
   d. antiinfective medications.

10. The fibrinolytic system functions by:

   a. allowing circulating platelets to aggregate and produce fibrin plugs.
   b. causing clot dissolution and formation of fibrin degradation products.
   c. converting prothrombin to thrombin.
   d. stimulating the intrinsic pathway.

11. Education of patients with AIDS and their significant others primarily includes:

   a. dehydration prevention through adequate intake.
   b. diarrhea control with medications.
   c. pain relief and comfort measures.
   d. understanding of disease transmission and the course of the disease.

12 A patient with severe thrombocytopenia is given:

   a. fresh frozen plasma.
   b. factor VIII cryoprecipitate.
   c. single-donor platelet products.
   d. absorbable gelatin sponge.

Matching—Key Terms

1. _____ Active immunity
2. _____ Antibody
3. _____ Anticoagulants
4. _____ Antigen
5. _____ Cellular immunity
6. _____ Cytokines
7. _____ DIC
8. _____ Epistaxis
9. _____ Hemarthrosis
10. _____ Hematochezia
11. _____ Hematopoiesis
12. _____ Humoral immunity
13. _____ Lymphoreticular system
14. _____ Passive immunity
15. _____ Procoagulants
16. _____ Purpura
17. _____ Reticulocytes
18. _____ Tissue anergy

a. Bleeding from the nose

b. Production of cytokines in response to foreign antigen

c. Cells and organs containing immunologically active cells

d. Factors enhancing clotting mechanisms

e. Any substance capable of stimulating an immune response

f. Occurs when the body actively produces cells and mediators, resulting in antigen destruction

g. Cell killer substances or mediators; secreted by WBCs

h. Production of antibodies in response to foreign proteins

i. Absence of a "wheal" response to an antigen; evidence of altered antibody capability

j. Occurs when antibodies to a specific disease are transferred from another person

k. Blood in a joint cavity

l. Development of the early blood cells in bone marrow or lymphoreticular organs

m. Immune globulin designed to destroy a specific antigen

n. Slightly immature erythrocytes

o. Large, mottled bruises

p. Bright red blood in stool

q. Also called "consumptive coagulopathy"

r. Factors inhibiting the clotting process

Matching—Blood Products

1. _____ Whole blood

2. _____ Red blood cells (RBCs)

3. _____ Washed RBCs (leukocyte-poor)

4. _____ Fresh frozen plasma

5. _____ Platelets

6. _____ Cryoprecipitate antihemophilic factor (AHF)

7. _____ Albumin

8. _____ Granulocytes

a. Plasma rich in clotting factors, platelets removed

b. Intravascular volume expander, increases osmotic pressure; prepared from plasma

c. RBCs, plasma, and stable clotting factors; restores volume and O_2-carrying capacity

d. RBCs without leukocytes and plasma proteins; restores volume and O_2-carrying capacity

e. Prepared by centrifugation or filtration; increases leukocyte level

f. RBCs from whole blood; restores volume and O_2-carrying capacity

g. Primarily factor VIII with fibrinogen and some factor XIII

h. Removed from whole blood; increases platelet count; improves hemostasis

PERSONALIZE IT!!

❖ Have you ever volunteered to donate blood? Are there any medical reasons why you are unable to donate? Do you believe that blood donation is a civic responsibility? Many people report actually feeling physically better after donating a unit of blood; all donors report a sense of personal satisfaction.

❖ A great deal of research is being done on the mind-body connection and its effects on the immune system. Can you describe any physiological manifestations of stress responses? Do you believe mental attitudes impact health?

❖ Many herbal preparations can affect bleeding tendencies by themselves or in combination with prescribed medications. If no information is available on your unit, it would be a worthwhile project to compile a reference sheet on these preparations.

CROSSWORD PUZZLE

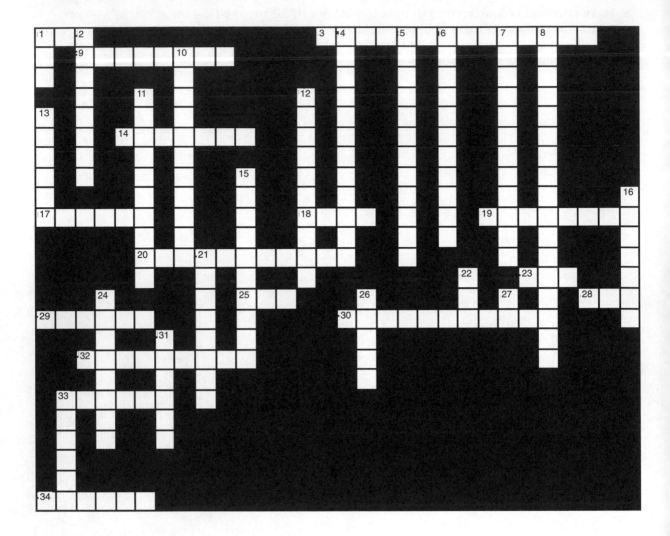

Across

1. Abbreviation for products produced when clots break down.
3. Presence of HIV antibodies seen 2 to 12 weeks postexposure.
9. Malignant disorder of WBCs.
14. Type of immunity mediated by B lymphocytes; involves antibody formation.
17. Absence of a response to antigens.
18. Abbreviation for activated partial thromboplastin time.
19. Cancer affecting the lymphocytes.
20. Cells that contain bactericidal substances.
23. Abbreviation for bone marrow transplant.
25. Most abundant immunoglobulin.
28. Abbreviation for the virus that causes AIDS.
29. _____ T cells stimulate B cells to differentiate and produce antibodies.
30. Cells essential for tumor immunity.
32. Cells that participate in allergic and inflammatory responses.
33. Immunity in which the body produces cells.
34. Bone _____ is the primary site of hematopoietic cell production.

Down

1. Abbreviation for fresh frozen plasma.
2. Another term for thrombocyte.
4. The primary component of these cells is hemoglobin.
5. Term for bleeding disorder.
6. Granulocytes responsible for phagocytosis.
7. Immature RBC.
8. Term used to describe someone with a risk for infection.
10. After maturation, these cells become "seek and destroy" scavengers.
11. Other name for white blood cells.
12. Formation of the platelet clot.
13. _____ comprises 55% of blood volume.
15. An example is HIV, RNA is transcribed into DNA.
16. Type of immunity that is passed on; temporary.
21. Ability to resist and fight infection.
22. Disorder of hemostasis in which clotting factors are "all used up" (abbreviation).
24. Type of anemia characterized by a failure of the marrow to produce any cells.
26. Breakdown of a clot.
27. Abbreviation for prothrombin time.
31. This organ, along with the liver, is essential for the clearance of RBCs.
33. Decrease in functional RBCs.

CONCEPT MAP

Mr. O., 76, is being treated in your unit for urosepsis. During your morning assessment, you notice bleeding around his Foley catheter and decreased urine output. Mr. O. seems confused, which is unusual for him at this time of the day. What disorder do you suspect, and what tests/treatments do you anticipate?

Assessment

Laboratory Findings

Nursing Diagnoses

Expected Medical Treatment

Nursing Interventions

Pathophysiology

Chapter 14

GASTROINTESTINAL ALTERATIONS

LEARNING OUTCOMES

- Understand the anatomy and physiology of the gastrointestinal system.
- Describe a general assessment of the gastrointestinal system.
- Discuss the nutritional assessment and therapies used for providing optimal nutrition.
- Compare the pathophysiology, assessment, nursing diagnoses, outcomes, and interventions for acute upper GI bleeding, acute pancreatitis, and hepatic failure.
- Formulate a plan of care for the patient with acute upper GI bleeding, acute pancreatitis, or hepatic failure.

TERMINOLOGY

- acini cells
- anabolism
- ascites
- asterixis
- basal metabolic rate (BMR)
- bilirubin
- catabolism
- cholecystokinin
- Chvostek's sign (hypocalcemia)
- chyme
- conjugated (direct) bilirubin
- encephalopathy
- gastric lavage
- gastric mucosal barrier
- gluconeogenesis
- glycogenesis
- glycogenolysis
- haustration

- hematemesis
- hematochezia
- hepatorenal syndrome
- histamine
- *H. pylori*
- hydrochloric acid
- intrinsic factor
- islets of Langerhans
- melena
- pancreatic alpha cells
- pancreatic beta cells
- pepsinogen
- peristalsis
- sclerotherapy
- splanchnic circulation
- total parenteral nutrition (TPN)
- Trousseau's sign (hypocalcemia)
- unconjugated (indirect) bilirubin

KEY POINTS

❖ Gastrointestinal Anatomy and Physiology

- The primary function of the alimentary or gastrointestinal tract and accessory organs is to provide the body with a continual supply of nutrients. This involves motility, digestion, and absorption.

- The gut wall is composed of multiple tissue layers:

  - Mucosa: innermost layer of tightly packed cells; forms a protective barrier. Goblet cells produce mucus.

    - Gastric mucosal barrier of stomach is impermeable to hydrochloric acid

  - Submucosa is composed of connective tissue, blood vessels, and nerve fibers

  - Muscular layer is next, then outer serosa with ANS innervation

- Oropharynx: Mastication; three pairs salivary glands. Saliva contains mucus and salivary amylase, a starch-digesting enzyme.

- Pharynx: Swallowing has three stages—oral, pharyngeal, and esophageal. Lower esophageal sphincter is not an anatomic sphincter, but prevents gastric acid reflux.

- Stomach regions are the cardia, fundus, body, antrum (greater curvature), and pylorus. The pyloric sphincter opens between the stomach and duodenum.

  - Food is mixed with gastric secretions to form chyme.

  - Gastric secretions are from mucosal cells and oxyntic and pyloric glands.

    - Oxyntic gland cells are mucous neck cells (mucus); peptic or chief cells (pepsinogen); and oxyntic, or parietal, cells (hydrochloric acid).

    - Intrinsic factor is produced by the parietal cells; it is necessary for absorption of B_{12} in the ileum.

    - Gastric fluid is also rich in sodium, potassium, and other electrolytes.

- Small intestine:

  - First 10 to 12 inches is the duodenum; pancreatic juices and bile empty into it. Brunner's glands secrete protective mucus. More than 50% of peptic ulcers occur here. Stomach acid stimulates the duodenum to produce the hormone secretin, which stimulates pancreatic secretions.

  - Next 7 to 8 feet are the jejunum, followed by 10 to 12 feet of ileum. Small pits called crypts of Lieberkuhn produce intestinal secretions (2000 ml/day). The ileocecal valve marks the beginning of the large intestine.

- Large intestine: Ascending, transverse and descending colon, and rectum. Functions are absorption of water and electrolytes from chyme and storage of fecal matter until defecation. Haustration is the characteristic contractile activity of the colon.

- Pancreas: Lies retroperitoneally in right and left upper quadrants of the abdomen. Functions include exocrine (digestive enzymes from acini) and endocrine (insulin and glucagon from beta and alpha cells, respectively, of islets of Langerhans).

- Liver: The largest internal organ, in upper right abdominal quadrant. Performs over 400 vascular, secretory, and metabolic functions.

- Vascular—Stores up to 400 ml of blood in the sinusoids. Hepatic vascular resistance is normally low. Kupffer's cells are extremely phagocytic; they remove bacteria and foreign material from the blood.

- Secretory—500 to 1000 ml of bile daily, which is stored in the gallbladder. Bilirubin, a metabolic end product of Hgb breakdown, is conjugated by the liver to prevent toxic effects. Most is secreted into bile.

- Metabolic—maintenance of normal blood glucose levels through glycogenesis, glycogenolysis, and gluconeogenesis. The liver produces all nonessential amino acids and all plasma proteins except gamma globulin. It is the site for conversion of excess carbohydrates and proteins to triglycerides; for production and removal of blood clotting factors, detoxification of drugs, and vitamin and mineral storage.

- Gallbladder: Stores and concentrates bile. Flow of bile into the duodenum is controlled by the sphincter of Oddi at the end of the common bile duct. The hormone cholecystokinin controls contraction of the gallbladder.

- Blood supply to abdominal organs is called the splanchnic circulation; receives approximately 33% of cardiac output.

- General assessment:

  - History includes any GI problems, pain, precipitating factors, prior surgeries, weight fluctuations, and medications.

  - Inspection and auscultation—Look for symmetry, pulsations, jaundice, masses; listen for bowel sounds or bruit.

  - Percussion and palpation—Percussed tympany predominates because of presence of gas. Palpate last; may cause pain or muscle spasm.

- Nutritional support should be considered early. Anabolism reflects a positive nitrogen balance; catabolism is a negative nitrogen balance and represents protein breakdown. Generally 25 calories per kg/day is sufficient with careful fluid balance.

  - Enteral nutrition in the form of special formulas is delivered into the GI tract orally or by means of nasogastric or other tube. Diarrhea and aspiration are possible complications. Blood glucose levels need monitoring until stabilized.

  - Total parenteral nutrition (TPN) is administered through a peripherally inserted central catheter or a central line; it contains all necessary nutrients for the patient's specific needs. Infection, fluid and electrolyte imbalance, osmotic diuresis, and sepsis are the major complications. Blood glucose is monitored every 6 hours.

❖ Acute Upper GI Bleed

- Peptic ulcer disease: Duodenal and gastric ulcers are the most common cause of upper GI bleeding.

  - Risk factors include alcohol, aspirin and nonsteroidal antiinflammatory drugs, smoking, genetic predisposition, and stress.

  - *Helicobacter pylori* (*H. pylori*) bacteria are often implicated; a double- or triple-agent therapy is often used as treatment.

- Stress ulcers are acute mucosal erosion associated with severe trauma, long-term sepsis, severe burns (Curling's ulcer), cranial or CNS disease (Cushing's ulcer), and long-term ingestion of irritating medications. They can result in small to massive hemorrhages.

- A Mallory-Weiss tear is an arterial bleed from a longitudinal tear in the gastroesophageal mucosa, often from long-term use of NSAIDS or aspiration or excessive alcohol intake. These make up 10% to 15% of bleeds and often resolve spontaneously.

- Esophageal varices: In chronic cirrhotic liver failure, portal hypertension leads to formation of collateral circulation, especially in submucosa of the esophagus and rectum, anterior abdomen, and the parietal peritoneum. These massively dilated submucosal veins (pressure > 10 mm Hg) are called varices. They cannot tolerate higher pressure and often bleed.

- Clinical presentation of upper GI bleed:

  - Hematemesis—bloody vomitus, either bright red (fresh) or "coffee ground" (older).

  - Melena—shiny, dark, foul-smelling stool or hematochezia; bright red blood passed rectally.

  - Signs of blood loss—restlessness, hypotension, dizziness, tachycardia, dyspnea, decreased LOC, decreased urine output, and hypovolemic shock.

- Nursing assessment:

  - First priority is to determine severity of blood loss.

  - Take frequent vital signs; watch for cool, clammy skin; monitor urine output and abdominal girth.

  - Hypotension is an advanced sign of shock.

- Medical assessment:

  - CBC—Hematocrit does not change significantly during first few hours. Clotting times are checked.

  - Electrolytes—Potassium and sodium may be lost because of vomiting. Glucose may be elevated. BUN and creatinine may be elevated. Calcium may be normal or elevated.

  - ABGs show respiratory alkalosis as a result of SNS effects and anxiety.

  - Liver function enzymes indicate prior disease.

  - Endoscopy is the procedure of choice for diagnosis of bleeding site.

- Nursing diagnoses include fluid volume deficit, anxiety, altered systemic tissue perfusion, impaired gas exchange, knowledge deficit (patient and family), and risk for aspiration. Later there is potential for fluid volume excess, altered electrolyte balance, and hepatic encephalopathy.

- Management involves hemodynamic stabilization, diagnosis of cause of bleeding, and supportive therapies.

  - Hemodynamic stabilization consists of colloids or crystalloids to restore vascular volume; then blood or blood products are transfused to improve oxygenation and coagulation. Supplemental O_2 is given.

    - One unit of packed RBCs usually increases Hgb value by 1 g/dl and the Hct value by 2% to 3%.

  - Bed rest is maintained with head of bed elevated; suctioning is performed as needed.

- Gastric lavage is a controversial therapy; it can indicate rapidity of the bleed, and it cleanses the stomach prior to endoscopy.

- Pharmacologic agents decrease gastric acid secretion or reduce its effects—antacids, H_2-histamine blockers, and mucosal barrier enhancers. However, it is thought that acid-reducing medications may increase the risk of nosocomial infections in intubated patients.

- Endoscopic therapies include sclerotherapy, the injection of a bleeding ulcer with a necrotizing agent; and thermal methods such as heater probe, laser coagulation, and electrocoagulation. Left lateral reverse Trendelenberg position helps prevent respiratory complications.

- Massive rebleeding may necessitate surgery to prevent death from exsanguination: gastric resections, Billroth I & II (to restore GI continuity), or vagotomy to decrease acid secretion.

- Postoperative nausea, vomiting, diarrhea and ileus are common, as are respiratory complications due to shallow breathing in response to incisional pain.

- Perforation is the major complication; symptoms include abrupt onset of abdominal pain followed by signs of peritonitis. Emergency surgery and antibiotic therapy are required.

- Variceal bleeds generally cause massive upper GI bleeding. Gastric lavage and endoscopy help with diagnosis; vasopressin (Pitressin) acts directly on GI smooth muscle as a vasoconstrictor but is also a diuretic and may induce water retention. Ocreotide is a somastatin derivative used for vasoconstriction, which has fewer side effects.

  - If vasopressin therapy doesn't stop the bleed, balloon tamponade (Sengstaken-Blakemore tube) is considered. On removal, the esophageal balloon must be deflated before the gastric balloon to prevent upward displacement and airway occlusion.

  - Other options include sclerotherapy, banding, transjugular intrahepatic portosystemic shunt, and portacaval shunts. Temporary increase in ascites occurs after these procedures. Patients are also at increased risk for encephalopathy after shunt procedures.

❖ Acute Pancreatitis

- Acute pancreatitis is a mild to severe acute inflammatory disease resulting from premature activation of pancreatic enzymes within the pancreas.

- 85% to 90% of cases are mild and self-limiting; severe cases have high mortality. Most common causes are alcohol ingestion and cholelithiasis (gallstones).

  - Common effects of all forms include hyperglycemia, hypoglycemia, and nutritional depletion. Severe abdominal pain often radiates to the back.

  - In severe acute hemorrhagic pancreatitis, look for Grey Turner's sign (bluish flank discoloration) or Cullen's sign (periumbilical discoloration).

  - Serum lipase and amylase tests are the best diagnostic indicators. CT and MRI help distinguish pancreatic pseudocyst, abscess or perforation, and biliary obstruction.

  - Acute respiratory and/or renal failure are major complications; coagulation abnormalities and cardiac failure can also accompany severe pancreatitis. The Ranson scale rates morbidity according to signs present in first 48 hours. Multisystem organ dysfunction syndrome may ensue.

- Nursing diagnoses and interventions are similar to general upper GI bleed. Nasogastric suction is generally required to suppress pancreatic exocrine secretions. Oral care and skin care around the NG tube are essential, as well as pain control. Morphine is now considered the first choice for analgesia.

❖ Hepatic Failure

- Hepatic failure can result from necrosis, cirrhosis, fatty liver, or decreased blood supply.

- Hepatitis is an acute inflammation of hepatocytes, generally of viral origin.

  - Hepatitis A—most common; oral-fecal route; usually mild

  - Hepatitis B—serum hepatitis; transmitted by blood and body fluids; can be chronic; higher chance of progression to fulminant disease.

  - Hepatitis C—transmitted by blood products and body fluids; usually mild; can be chronic

  - Hepatitis D—always with hepatitis B; transmitted by blood and body fluids; can be chronic

  - Hepatitis E—epidemic in underdeveloped countries; fecal-oral route; not chronic

- Symptoms of hepatitis include jaundice, brown urine, loss of appetite, nausea, vomiting, fever, weakness and chills.

- Nursing diagnoses include activity intolerance, altered nutrition, risk for infection, and risk for altered thought processes. There is no definitive treatment; rest and nutritional support are essential.

- When caring for a patient with hepatitis, special precautions include use of disposable patient care items, private room and bathroom, gowns and gloves, and double bagging or labeling linen and contaminated equipment.

- Cirrhosis refers to irreversible fibrotic changes, which result from liver lobule compression by inflammation and necrosis. The four types are alcoholic (Laënnec's), biliary, cardiac, and postnecrotic.

- Fatty liver refers to an accumulation of excessive fats in the liver, also often caused by alcohol abuse. Other causes are obesity, diabetes, hepatic resection, starvation, and TPN.

- Functional sequelae of liver disease:

  - Portal hypertension—causes hyperdynamic circulation and formation of esophageal or gastric varices and splenomegaly.

  - Impaired metabolic processes—unstable glucose levels; fatigue; fatty liver; decreased synthesis and removal of clotting factors; decreased metabolism of vitamins and iron; decreased detoxification functions; loss of Kupffer cell activity increases risk of infection.

  - Impairment of bile production and flow—increased serum bilirubin levels and resultant jaundice.

- Diagnostics include liver function lab tests, liver biopsy, and ultrasound studies of bile flow.

- Treatments focus on maintaining hemodynamic stability, administration of vasoactive drugs and fluids, and minimizing complications. Liver transplantation is an option in severe cases.

- Ascites is common; breathing is impaired because of upward pressure on the diaphragm. It is managed with bed rest, low-sodium diet, fluid restriction, diuretic therapy, and paracentesis.

- Portal systemic (hepatic) encephalopathy is progressive damage to the CNS causing altered LOC, asterixis, extreme confusion, and ultimately coma. Abnormal ammonia levels are thought to be a factor, so protein intake is limited. Neomycin and lactulose are medications that reduce bacterial breakdown of protein in the bowel, thus reducing ammonia production.

- Hepatorenal syndrome is acute renal failure that occurs with liver failure and generally has a poor prognosis.

REVIEW QUESTIONS

True/False

1. **T F** Intrinsic factor is secreted only by the parietal cells of the stomach.

2. **T F** Chyme is secreted only by the small intestine.

3. **T F** Pepsin is active only in an environment with pH greater than 6.0.

4. **T F** Vitamin B_{12} is absorbed in the proximal ileum in the presence of intrinsic factor.

5. **T F** Blood is supplied to the liver by the hepatic artery and the portal vein.

6. **T F** Approximately 500 to 1000 ml of bile are produced by the liver daily.

7. **T F** The GI system receives the largest single percentage of the cardiac output.

8. **T F** A Mallory-Weiss tear usually occurs in the duodenal area.

9. **T F** Prostaglandins are helpful in protecting the musocal barrier.

10. **T F** The Minnesota tube and the Sengstaken-Blakemore tube are types of balloon tamponade used in esophageal varices when vasopressin therapy has failed.

Multiple Choice

1. A sympathetic response could exacerbate a duodenal ulcer because of its inhibitory effects on:

   a. gastrin.
   b. Brunner's glands.
   c. parietal cells.
   d. pepsin.

2. A mechanism of the liver that breaks down stored glycogen during episodes of hypoglycemia is:

   a. conjugation.
   b. gluconeogenesis.
   c. glycogenesis.
   d. glycogenolysis.

3. Treatment of bleeding ulcers can include sclerotherapy and thermal endoscopic methods. The purpose of these therapies is to:

   a. delay surgery for patients requiring up to 8 pints of blood.
   b. prevent ARDS as a result of exposure to fatty substances.
   c. prevent exsanguination in the case of perforation.
   d. tamponade the vessel to stop active bleeding.

4. Death during the first two weeks of acute pancreatitis is usually the result of:

   a. ARDS and acute renal failure.
   b. disseminated intravascular coagulation or GI bleeding.
   c. hypocalcemia and hyperlipidemia.
   d. pancreatic pseudocysts.

5. Clinical symptoms of pancreatitis can mimic other GI diseases. The most significant lab test(s) in the differential diagnosis of pancreatitis is:

   a. blood serum triglycerides.
   b. partial thromboplastin time.
   c. serum lipase and amylase.
   d. total bilirubin.

6. What diet is recommended for the patient who has hepatitis and is experiencing loss of appetite, nausea, and vomiting?

   a. High fat, low protein
   b. High protein, low carbohydrate
   c. Low fat, high protein
   d. Low protein, high carbohydrate

7. Important teaching for patients who have hepatitis and their family members includes:

   a. counseling about sexual transmission.
   b. handwashing and personal hygiene techniques.
   c. hepatitis B screening for pregnant women and HIV-positive patients.
   d. all of the above.

8. Patients in hepatic failure may experience gram-negative sepsis as a result of damage to which cells?

   a. Acini cells
   b. Alpha cells
   c. Beta cells
   d. Kupffer's cells

9. A patient with acute pancreatitis should be monitored for:

   a. hypercalcemia.
   b. hypocalcemia.
   c. hyperkalemia.
   d. neutropenia.

10. The normal volume of secretions processed by the GI tract in a 24-hour period is approximately:

   a. 100–1000 ml.
   b. 2000–4000 ml.
   c. 4000–10,000 ml.
   d. 10,000–15,000 ml.

11. Vasopressin is administered via infusion pump at a rate of 0.2–0.4 U/min into a central line. This synthetic hormone acts by:

    a. vasoconstriction to decrease bleeding.
    b. increasing peripheral circulation.
    c. increasing renal flow.
    d. reducing water retention.

12. *Helicobacter pylori* bacteria are suspected in the development of:

    a. hepatic encephalopathy.
    b. hepatitis.
    c. pancreatitis.
    d. peptic ulcers.

Matching—Key Terms

1. _____ Secretin
2. _____ Cholecystikinin
3. _____ Gastrin
4. _____ Pepsinogen
5. _____ Trypsinogen
6. _____ Amylase
7. _____ Vasopressin
8. _____ Glucagon
9. _____ Histamine
10. _____ Bilirubin

a. secreted in an inactive form to prevent pancreatic autodigestion

b. stimulates contraction of gallbladder and secretion of pancreatic enzymes

c. the salivary type is a starch-digesting enzyme

d. a pigment; a metabolic end-product of Hgb break down

e. secreted by alpha cells of the pancreas

f. synthetic antidiuretic hormone

g. stimulates bicarbonate production in the liver and pancreas

h. secreted by peptic (chief) cells

i. stimulates release of gastrin and hydrochloric acid

j. stimulates secretory and mechanical activity of the stomach

PERSONALIZE IT!!

❖ Mrs. J., 60, was hospitalized for an upper GI bleed, which was attributed to long-term use of NSAIDS for her arthritic pain. She is 20 pounds overweight, and she reports general stiffness and joint pain. Would you consider recommending that she consult with her physician about an exercise plan (after recovery)? Do you think addition of an antiulcer medication is a good solution?

❖ Some GI bleeds occur as a result of conditions such as Crohn's disease, ulcerative colitis, or even long-term eating disorders. Some require ostomy surgery. Does your unit have an updated list of support groups? If not, compile one, starting with organizations like Alcoholics Anonymous, Crohn's and Colitis Foundation of America, and United Ostomy Association. These and many more can be accessed via the Internet.

CROSSWORD PUZZLE

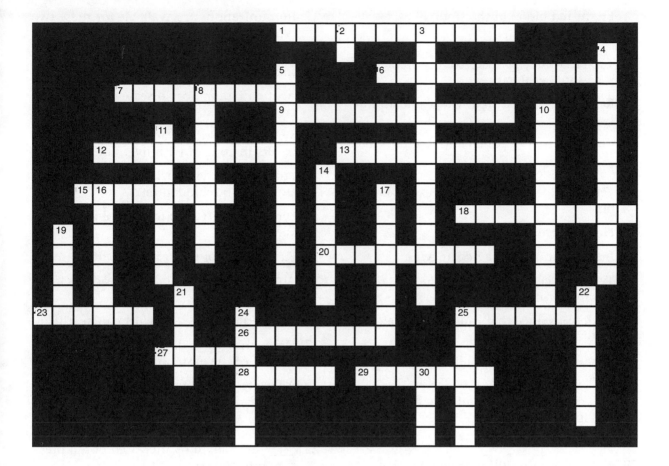

Across

1. Bright red blood in the stool.

6. Calcium level < 8 mg/dl.

7. Tube that may be inserted to stop bleeding esophageal varices.

9. Removal of ascitic fluid via needle aspiration.

12. Complication of pancreatitis.

13. Bloody vomitus.

15. Yellow coloring of skin from excess bilirubin.

18. Flapping tremors.

20. Inflammation of the hepatocytes.

23. Type of ulcer of the gastric mucosa commonly occurring in ICUs.

25. Toxic substance that causes encephalopathy.

26. Organ that secretes insulin and glucagons.

27. _____ liver is an accumulation of excess fats in the liver.

28. Largest internal organ of the body.

29. Type of ulcer resulting from a break in the mucosa of the stomach.

Down

2. Immunizations are available for these two types of hepatitis.

3. Condition caused by substances that are toxic to the liver.

4. Acute inflammatory disease of the pancreas.

5. Syndrome in which acute renal failure occurs in concert with liver failure.

8. Procedure for visualizing the inside of the stomach and duodenum.

10. Synthetic ADH used to control bleeding varices.

11. First section of the small intestine.

14. Abuse of this substance can lead to cirrhosis.

16. Elevated enzyme seen with pancreatitis.

17. Drugs that act as direct buffers to increase the pH of the gastric mucosa.

19. A LeVeen _____ helps to relieve ascites.

21. Hepatitis A is spread through the ___-oral route.

22. _____ are caused by increased portal pressure into the esophagus.

24. Bacteria known to cause ulcers (abbreviation).

25. Accumulation of fluid in the peritoneum.

30. Abbreviation for procedure for reducing portal pressure.

CONCEPT MAP

Complete a comprehensive data map for Mr. G., a 64-year-old man admitted with exertional dyspnea, muscle weakness and fatigue, bruising, urticaria, jaundiced sclera, and complaints of "stomach trouble." Mr. G.'s abdomen is distended even though he reports repeated vomiting for the past 12 hours, with "some bright red blood present." He admits to a history of alcohol abuse.

Client Medical Diagnosis

Laboratory Studies

Pertinent History

Predisposing Factors of the Diagnosis

Diagnostic Studies

Prioritized Problem List

Supportive Measures

Definitive Treatment
(possible prescribed meds, treatments, IV fluids)

Chapter 15

ENDOCRINE ALTERATIONS

LEARNING OUTCOMES

- Identify disorders resulting from hormones secreted by the pancreas and adrenal, thyroid, and posterior pituitary glands.
- Describe the feedback mechanisms for regulation of cortisol, antidiuretic hormone, thyroid hormone, and insulin.
- Compare pathophysiology, assessment, nursing diagnoses, outcomes, and interventions for hyperglycemic crisis, hypoglycemic crisis, adrenal crisis, thyroid storm, myxedema coma, diabetes insipidus, and the syndrome of inappropriate antidiuretic hormone secretion.
- Compare and contrast diabetic ketoacidosis and hyperosmolar hyperglycemic nonketotic coma.
- Formulate plans of care for patients with endocrine alterations.

TERMINOLOGY

- Addison's disease
- adrenocorticotropic hormone (ACTH)
- antidiuretic hormone (ADH)
- arginine vasopressin
- corticotropin-releasing hormone (CRH)
- diabetes insipidus (DI)
- diabetic ketoacidosis (DKA)
- exophthalmos
- Grave's disease
- hyperosmolar hyperglycemic nonketotic coma (HHNC)

- ketosis
- Kussmaul's respiration
- lipolysis
- myxedema coma
- negative feedback
- positive feedback
- syndrome of inappropriate antidiuretic hormone (SIADH) secretion
- thyroxine (T_4)
- triiodothyronine (T_3)
- thyroid storm

KEY POINTS

❖ The Endocrine System

- The endocrine system is composed of ductless, highly vascular glands, which produce hormones that regulate bodily functions in conjunction with the nervous system. The hypothalamus (a neuroendocrine organ) conveys inhibiting and releasing hormones to the pituitary, which responds to varying hormone levels through a feedback control mechanism.

  - Positive feedback systems stimulate hormone release when levels are low.

  - Negative feedback systems inhibit hormone release when levels are high.

  - Other primary endocrine organs are the pancreas, adrenal glands, and thyroid gland.

❖ Pancreatic Endocrine Emergencies

- Insulin is released by beta cells in the islets of Langerhans primarily in response to increased serum glucose levels. It is necessary for uptake of glucose by most body cells; without it, glucose cannot enter the cells and accumulates in the blood (hyperglycemia), causing cells to starve. With excess insulin, blood glucose levels decrease and the CNS is affected, with changes in LOC. Diabetes mellitus (DM) is a metabolic disease of glucose imbalance, caused by alteration in insulin secretion, action, or both.

  - Type 1 (immune-mediated) is an absolute insulin deficiency; often leads to ketoacidosis.

  - Type 2 involves insulin resistance with a secretory defect; it is a relative insulin deficiency and is more prevalent.

- Diabetic ketoacidosis (DKA) is an endocrine emergency resulting from a sustained relative or absolute insulin deficiency. Often it is the first indication for a new diagnosis of DM. In known insulin-dependent diabetics, it can result from infections and severe stress states that require higher insulin supply. It generally develops rapidly.

  - Insufficient insulin hinders cellular uptake of glucose, causing it to accumulate in the blood. This produces an osmotic gradient between intracellular and extracellular spaces causing fluid to move out of the cells (cellular dehydration).

  - The liver responds to the starving cells by converting glycogen to glucose and nitrogen, but without insulin they cannot be used, further increasing serum blood glucose and blood urea nitrogen (BUN). Intracellular potassium is lost.

  - Osmotic diuresis of glucose through the kidneys (glycosuria) leads to urinary losses of water, sodium, potassium, magnesium, calcium, and phosphorus. Serum osmolarity increases, worsening dehydration. The GFR then decreases because of fluid volume deficits; further hyperosmolarity results.

  - Meanwhile, the absolute insulin deficiency causes fat breakdown (lipolysis) into glycerol and fatty acids, which accumulate in the liver and are broken down into ketone acids. In the blood, H^+ ions dissociate from the ketones and bicarbonate buffering is impaired, leading to metabolic acidosis.

  - As acidosis increases, the respiratory system attempts to blow off excess CO_2 with deep, rapid breathing (Kussmaul's respiration). Worsening dehydration causes decreased perfusion to core organs, causing hypoxemia and worsening lactic acidosis.

- This deadly cycle of diminished glucose excretion and increasing blood glucose levels produces worsening hyperosmolarity and dehydration and, in combination with worsening acidosis, eventually leads to shock, coma, and death.

- Hyperosmotic hyperglycemic nonketotic coma (HHNC) is also a pancreatic emergency, characterized by extreme hyperglycemia, hyperosmolarity, and severe dehydration, but lower levels of free fatty acids than in DKA and thus a lack of ketosis.

  - The cycle of cellular dehydration and increasing hyperosmolarity are generally more severe than in DKA because HHNC develops insidiously over weeks or months.

  - Mortality rates are higher in HHNC because of the fact that patients are profoundly dehydrated and hyperosmolar by the time they seek medical treatment. More of these patients are also elderly with comorbid conditions.

  - HHNC often occurs in newly diagnosed type 2 diabetics, after high-calorie parenteral or enteral feedings, or as a result of certain medications.

- Clinical presentation of DKA and HHNK:

  - Polydipsia, polyuria, and polyphagia (in elderly, less polydipsia)

  - Signs of intravascular dehydration: hypotension, tachycardia, warm dry skin, dry mucous membranes, loss of skin turgor, and sunken eyeballs.

  - Vomiting, decreasing urine output

  - Weakness and anorexia

  - Clear lung fields

  - Altered LOC: restlessness, confusion, agitation, somnolence, coma

  - Decreased deep tendon reflexes; seizures

- DKA features: history of type 1 DM; rapid onset; nausea and vomiting; Kussmaul's respirations; acetone (fruity) breath; pH < 7.30 and decreased bicarbonate; blood glucose levels 600–800 mg/dl; ketone acids present in blood and urine; often hyperkalemic.

- HHNC features: history of type 2 DM; more often elderly; slow onset; shallow respirations; more profound LOC changes; blood glucose levels > 1000 mg/dl; pH > 7.30; no ketosis; often hypernatremic

- Nursing diagnoses for both DKA and HHNC include fluid volume deficit, ineffective breathing pattern, sensory/perceptual alterations, altered electrolyte balance, altered acid-base balance, and knowledge deficit.

- Interventions

  - ABCs, O_2, oral airways, ventilatory support if needed.

  - Monitor for hypovolemic shock; fluid replacement (3–4 L in DKA, up to 10 L in HHNC) of NS initially until BP normalizes, then hypotonic saline. Half of the estimated fluid deficit is replaced in the first 8 hours, the second half over the next 16 hours.

  - Insulin replacement is the definitive therapy. Low-dose continuous infusion provides a gradual decrease in serum glucose. As levels approach 300 mg/dl, 5% glucose is added to replacement fluid.

    - Prevents hypoglycemia with continued insulin infusion and prevents cerebral edema

- Frequent glucose level monitoring is essential, every 1–2 hours, using one method consistently. Later monitoring is done at 6- to 8-hour intervals.

- Monitor electrolytes with individualized replacement therapy.

- Acidosis (DKA) is not treated with bicarbonate until pH is 7.10 or less.

- ABGs are performed frequently.

- Patient and family education—An effective teaching plan can help prevent recurrence, especially of DKA. Teaching includes understanding the disease, recognizing early signs, treatments for control, record keeping, and anticipating situations of increased insulin requirements.

- Hypoglycemia is a state of decreased blood glucose level to 45–60 mg/dl or less (insulin shock). Headache, irritability, and dizziness are early LOC changes; prolonged hypoglycemia can lead to irreversible damage and coma.

  - Occurs with inconsistent rotation of insulin injection sites, delayed meals or missed snacks, interrupted tube feedings, weight loss, strenuous exercise without increased caloric intake, drug interactions, or any mechanism associated with excess of insulin supply in relation to the need.

  - The sympathetic nervous system is activated by falling glucose levels, resulting in release of epinephrine. Tachycardia, diaphoresis, pallor, and dilated pupils result along with general tremulousness and weakness.

  - Treatment is administration of 10–20 g of carbohydrate orally, or high concentration IV glucose or glucagon injection IM in emergent situations. Glucose levels are checked 15 to 30 minutes after treatment and repeated as necessary.

  - ECG and electrolyte monitoring are also important.

  - Patient education is crucial for prevention.

❖ Acute Adrenal Crisis

- The adrenal medulla mainly secretes catecholamines; the adrenal cortex secretes corticosteroids, adrenal androgens, and estrogen. Insufficient secretion by the adrenal cortex of glucocorticoids (cortisol) and/or mineralcorticoids (aldosterone) can result in adrenal crisis, affecting the body's defense mechanisms and stress response.

  - Corticotropin-releasing hormone (CRH) from the hypothalamus stimulates the pituitary to produce adrenocorticotropic hormone (ACTH), which stimulates cortisol production by the adrenal cortex.

    - Cortisol levels peak in the morning and are lowest around midnight. In stress situations, cortisol levels may increase up to 10 times the normal value. Cortisol increases blood glucose levels by promoting the breakdown of glycogen and gluconeogenesis, increases lipolysis and free fatty acid production, increases protein degradation, and inhibits the inflammatory and immune responses.

  - Aldosterone synthesis is regulated mainly by the renin-angiotensin system. It acts in the kidneys to increase sodium ion reabsorption and increases potassium and hydrogen ion excretion. An osmotic gradient across the renal tubular membrane results, activating antidiuretic hormone (ADH), which causes water to be reabsorbed with sodium.

- Acute adrenal crisis refers to an absolute or relative lack of cortisol and aldosterone.

  - Cortisol deficiency results in decreases in glucose production, protein and fat metabolism, appetite, intestinal motility, vascular tone and catecholamine effects. Stress conditions for a person with reduced cortisol can lead to profound shock.

  - Aldosterone deficiency results in decreases in sodium and water retention, and circulating volume, as well as increases in potassium and H+ ion reabsorption.

- Primary mechanisms cause destruction of the adrenal gland and result in Addison's disease, with decreases in both cortisol and aldosterone. Some are autoimmune destruction, infection, hemorrhagic, and granulomatous infiltration.

- Secondary mechanisms interfere with ACTH secretion or suppress corticosteroid production, generally resulting in glucocorticoid deficiency only. They include long-term steroid use (most common), and pituitary and hypothalamic disorders. Chronic steroid use suppresses the normal CRH-ACTH-adrenal feedback systems.

  - Many diseases (including COPD, SLE, asthma, and rheumatoid arthritis) are treated with corticosteroids, resulting in adrenal suppression.

  - Some drugs used to treat AIDS (trimethoprim and ketoconazole) suppress adrenal function, increasing the risk of acute adrenal crisis.

- Assessment includes drug, illness, and family histories; nutritional status; fatigue, dizziness, salt craving; low blood glucose levels unresponsive to therapy.

  - Headache, extreme fatigue, severe weakness are neurological signs. Cardiovascular signs are related to hypovolemia, decreased vascular tone, and hyperkalemia (ECG changes). Weak, rapid pulse, orthostatic hypotension, and cold pale skin are seen. Decreased CO can lead to hemodynamic collapse and shock.

  - Urine output decreases. Hyperpigmentation of mucous membranes, scar tissue, and skin over joints is common.

  - Labs show hypoglycemia, hyponatremia, hyperkalemia, increased BUN, and metabolic acidosis. Diagnosis is by plasma cortisol levels, which should be higher during stress.

- Nursing diagnoses include fluid volume deficit, altered perfusion, activity intolerance, altered nutrition and thought processes, and knowledge deficit.

- Interventions include fluid and electrolyte replacement (5% dextrose and NS), replacement of hormones (dexamethasone, Decadron, Solu-Cortef) and treatment of the underlying condition.

- Patient teaching is the key to prevention; patients should know when increased steroid doses are called for, and how to taper off from high dosages instead of an abrupt decrease.

❖ Thyroid Crises

- Thyroid hormones thyroxine (T_4) and triiodothyronine (T_3) are secreted by the thyroid gland under the influence of the pituitary gland via secretion of thyroid-stimulating hormone (TSH). They affect the metabolic functions of all body systems.

  - T_4 accounts for 90% of circulating thyroid hormone, but half of thyroid activity is from T_3

- T_3 is five times more potent and faster-acting; it is produced by conversion from T_4 in nonthyroid tissue

- T_3 and T_4 are highly bound to globulin, T_4-binding prealbumin, and albumin. Only the unbound fraction is biologically active.

- Excess thyroid hormones stimulate cellular energy production, leading to excessive thermal energy and fever. A hyperdynamic, hypermetabolic state disrupts many major body functions. Hyperthyroidism leads to weight loss, general muscle wasting, fatigue, thin skin, fine hair, splenomegaly, increased cardiac contractility and output, and ophthalmic disturbances (lid lag, exophthalmos). Symptoms may be masked in the elderly.

  - Toxic diffuse goiter (Graves' disease) is the most common. Possibly of autoimmune origin, it most commonly affects women aged 30–40. Inflammation and enlargement of the thyroid gland are present.

  - Toxic multinodular goiter is the second most common cause of hyperthyroidism. Affects mostly women aged 40–70.

  - Toxic uninodular goiter is less common.

- Thyroid storm is a life-threatening condition resulting from a rapid rise in free thyroid levels. Possible causes are a sudden change in levels of binding proteins (postoperatively), decreased binding affinity, or saturation of hormone-binding capacity leading to rapid release of thyroid hormones into the bloodstream (as from radioactive iodine treatment, post-thyroid surgery, or thyroid hormone overdose).

  - Thyroid storm usually occurs in untreated or undertreated hyperthyroidism, and as a result of added stressors (surgery, trauma, infection, emotional stress). Onset is abrupt, with severe fever, marked tachycardia, tremors, agitation, delirium, stupor, and coma. High mortality rate if untreated.

    - Increased protein catabolism causes severe muscle weakness. Stimulation of catecholamines causes a hyperdynamic heart, which can lead to decreasing CO and heart failure as muscles weaken. Common dysrhythmias include PACs, atrial fibrillation, and atrial flutter. Skin is warm, moist, and pink

    - Weakness causes respiratory inefficiency and CO_2 retention. Abdominal pain, nausea, vomiting, and diarrhea may be present.

  - Diagnostics include T_3 and T_4 levels, resin T_3 uptake (indirect measure of free T_4 levels). All are elevated in hyperthyroidism and may not be significantly different in thyroid storm.

  - Nursing diagnoses for thyroid storm include decreased cardiac output, hyperthermia, ineffective breathing pattern, altered nutrition, activity intolerance, altered thought processes, impaired skin integrity, and knowledge deficit.

  - Interventions include drugs to inhibit thyroid hormone biosynthesis (propylthiouracil [PTU], methimazole), but both are administered by oral route only and lack immediate effect. Beta blockers (propranolol, esmolol, atenolol) act rapidly to block peripheral effects of thyroid hormones; they decrease heart rate and CO and diminish supraventricular dysrhythmias.

    - Other slower-acting drugs include iodide agents, lithium carbonate, guanethidine, and reserpine.

    - Support measures include hydration, external cooling measures, stress doses of glucocorticoids, digoxin for patients with CHF, high-calorie, high-protein diets, and if necessary, dialysis and plasmapheresis.

- • Patient and family education include understanding of disease process, medication therapy, and situations requiring medical assistance.

- • Hypothyroidism:

  - • Low levels of thyroid hormones also disrupt the normal physiology of most body systems. Hypothyroidism commonly results from primary disease states such as autoimmune disorder (Hashimoto's thyroiditis), radiation treatment of Graves' disease, or thyroidectomy without sufficient hormone replacement. Secondary disease is most often due to pituitary tumor; tertiary to hypothalamic injury or disease.

    - • Early signs are fatigue, weakness, muscle cramps, and cold intolerance; symptoms are related to mucinous edema. Depression, lethargy, and personality changes occur with long-term disease.

    - • Cardiac, respiratory, and GI function are all diminished. Fluid retention and decreased metabolic rate result in weight gain and ascites. Skin is dry and cool; hair is coarse; tongue may be enlarged.

  - • Myxedma coma is a life-threatening condition related to severely low levels of thyroid hormone. It develops slowly in already hypothroid patients and is a magnification of the hypodynamic, hypometabolic state. It occurs most often in elderly females; mortality rates are high due to underlying illnesses.

    - • Presenting symptoms are slowed mentation, hypothermia, distant heart sounds, bradycardia, pericardial effusion, depressed respirations, decreased tendon reflexes, mucinous edema, coarse dry skin, and brittle hair.

    - • Lab values show low serum T_4, T_3, and resin T_3 uptake levels. In primary disease, TSH levels are high. In secondary or tertiary disease, TSH is inappropriately normal or low. Hyponatremia and low cortisol levels may occur.

  - • Nursing diagnoses include fluid volume excess, decreased CO, hypothermia, altered thought processes, ineffective breathing pattern, risk for injury, activity intolerance, altered nutrition, and knowledge deficit.

  - • Interventions include thyroid hormone replacement (levothyroxine sodium [most common] or liothyronine sodium), cautious volume expansion if hypotensive, or fluid restriction if hyponatremic. Passive methods (blankets) are supplied for hypothermia to prevent peripheral vasodilation and circulatory collapse. Supplemental O_2 and ventilatory support are given as needed; drugs, especially narcotics and sedatives, must be administered cautiously because of hypermetabolic state.

  - • Patient education is similar to teaching for hyperthyroidism.

- ❖ Antidiuretic Hormone (ADH) Disorders

  - • ADH (also called arginine vasopressin) is produced in the hypothalamus, stored in the posterior pituitary, and released in response to changes in extracellular osmolality, circulating volume, and blood pressure. Once released, ADH acts on the renal distal and collecting tubules to cause water reabsorption.

    - • ADH can also be released in response to stress, trauma, hypoxia, pain, or anxiety.

  - • Diabetes insipidus (DI) refers to impaired renal conservation of water and polyuria (> 3 L in 24 hours). If the thirst center remains intact, the patient can maintain fluid volume; otherwise, severe dehydration ensues.

- Types of DI:

  - Neurogenic DI (ADH deficiency)—Result of disruption of neural pathways involved in ADH production, synthesis, or release. Primary cause is traumatic injury to posterior pituitary or hypothalamus (trauma or surgery).

  - Nephrogenic DI (ADH insensitivity)—Kidneys are unable to respond to ADH. Usually a result of chronic renal disease, drugs, or other permanent kidney damage.

  - Secondary DI results from excessive water intake; can result from thirst regulation disorder, cognitive dysfunction (mental illness), or excess IV fluid administration.

- Symptoms of DI include polyuria (5–40 L in 24 hours), which may result in signs of hypovolemia (hypotension, decreased turgor, dry mucous membranes, tachycardia, weight loss, low CVP and pulmonary artery occlusion pressure). Decreased cerebral perfusion, cerebral dehydration, and hypernatremia cause neurological changes (confusion, restlessness, lethargy, seizures).

- Lab results show low urine osmolality, decreased urine specific gravity, but high serum osmolality. BUN and creatinine are elevated as a result of hemoconcentration. Plasma ADH is decreased in neurogenic DI, increased in nephrogenic DI, and normal in secondary DI. Other tests further differentiate etiology.

- Nursing diagnoses include fluid volume deficit and altered thought processes.

- Interventions are based on identification of underlying cause. Fluid replacement is provided according to urine loss and electrolyte status. Frequent VS and neuro checks; I&O, daily weights, ECG, urine specific gravity are all monitored. Breath sounds are closely monitored to prevent fluid overload.

  - Neurogenic DI is treated mainly with exogenous ADH (desmopressin); aqueous vasopressin and lysine vasopressin can also be used, but these have more vasoconstrictive effects. Overtreatment can produce water overload.

  - Nephrogenic DI is treated with solute restriction and thiazide diuretics.

  - Secondary DI is treated with water restriction and treatment of underlying disorders.

- Syndrome of inappropriate antidiuretic hormone (SIADH) secretion occurs when the body produces excess ADH unrelated to plasma osmolality, resulting in inability to secrete a dilute urine, fluid retention, and dilutional hyponatremia.

  - Causes of SIADH:

    - The most common cause is malignancy, especially bronchogenic carcinoma. Pancreatic, duodenal, and Hodgkin's lymphoma also can produce SIADH.

    - Nonmalignant pulmonary conditions such as TB, pneumonia, lung abscess, and COPD can cause SIADH.

    - CNS disorders such as head injury, infection, bleeds, and CVA are also causes. Medications—antineoplastics, anesthetics, anticonvulsants, oral hypoglycemics, narcotics, and barbiturates—are associated with SIADH.

- The clinical picture is water intoxication, related to severity of the hyponatremia and hypoosmolality. CNS response can be confusion, restlessness, seizures, and coma due to cerebral edema and increasing ICP. Nausea and vomiting, hypertension, dyspnea, and frothy pink sputum are often seen.

- Labs show hyponatremia and hypoosmolality in the presence of inappropriately concentrated urine with high sodium content.

- A water load test may be done to confirm etiology of the hyponatremia.

- Nursing diagnoses include fluid volume excess and altered thought processes.

- Interventions for mild to moderate cases (serum Na^+ 125–135 mEq/ml) are fluid restriction to 800–1000 ml/day, with liberal dietary salt and protein intake. In severe symptomatic cases (coma, seizures, Na^+ < 110 mEq/ml) hypertonic saline (3% or 5%), 200–300 ml is given over several hours with fluid intake restricted to 500 ml/day.

    - Hypertonic saline must be administered slowly to prevent demyelinization of nerves, cerebral edema, and seizures. Sodium levels are raised only to 120 mEq/ml or lower if symptoms resolve.

    - For irreversible conditions (such as malignancy), demeclocycline is used (an antibiotic that decreases renal responsiveness to ADH). Urea and lithium carbonate are also sometimes used.

    - The safest method for treating chronic hyponatremia is use of a loop diuretic with increased salt and potassium intake.

- SIADH may not be preventable, so recognizing at-risk populations and early detection and treatment are essential. Patient education includes early signs and symptoms, importance of fluid restriction, medication therapy, and daily weights.

REVIEW QUESTIONS

Multiple Choice

1. Poyldipsia, poyluria, abdominal pain, nausea, and "fruity" breath are typical findings in:

    a. Addison's disease.
    b. DKA.
    c. HHNC.
    d. myxedema coma.

2. Kussmaul's respiration, the rapid deep breathing seen in DKA, is the body's effort to rid itself of:

    a. bicarbonate.
    b. carbonic acid.
    c. lactic acid.
    d. ketone acid.

3. In HHNC, laboratory results are similar to those in DKA, but with three major exceptions. What do you expect to see in HHNC?

    a. Higher serum glucose, higher osmolality, and greater ketosis.
    b. Higher serum glucose, higher osmolality, and milder ketosis.
    c. Lower serum glucose, lower osmolality, and greater ketosis.
    d. Lower serum glucose, lower osmolality, and milder ketosis.

4. Cortisol is released in response to:

    a. anterior pituitary release of ACTH.
    b. decreased plasma sodium.
    c. increased blood glucose.
    d. renin-angiotensin system.

5. The hypothyroid state in secondary hypothyroidism is often caused by:

    a. age-related changes.
    b. congenital defects.
    c. destruction of the thyroid by radiation.
    d. pituitary gland dysfunction.

6. Assessment findings for a patient who is in myxedema coma include:

    a. nervousness, increased T_4, crackles, increased respirations.
    b. hypotension, tachycardia, polydipsia, temperature 102° F.
    c. lethargy, edema, swollen tongue, abdominal distention.
    d. weight gain, seizures, dark yellow urine, frothy pink sputum.

7. Mr. Roberts underwent thyroidectomy surgery five years ago. Recently his wife suffered a stroke; he is working part-time in order to care for her and reports he cannot afford his medications. What electrolyte imbalance would you expect to see?

   a. Hypernatremia
   b. Hyperglycemia
   c. Hyponatremia
   d. Metabolic alkalosis

8. In primary adrenal insufficiency, serum levels of all of the following are elevated *except*:

   a. calcium.
   b. potassium.
   c. sodium.
   d. BUN.

9. Mechanisms for development of diabetes insipidus include all *except*:

   a. ADH deficiency.
   b. ADH insensitivity.
   c. excessive water intake.
   d. water deprivation.

10. Signs of SIADH include which of the following?

   a. Hypernatremia
   b. Increased serum osmolality
   c. Increased urine osmolality
   d. Decreased water retention

Matching—Symptom : Hormone Level

1. _____ Diabetes insipidus

2. _____ Thyroid crisis (storm)

3. _____ Type 2 diabetes mellitus

4. _____ Cushing's syndrome

5. _____ SIADH

6. _____ Myxedema coma

7. _____ Acute adrenal crisis

8. _____ Hypoglycemia

a. Hypersecretion of ADH

b. Hypersecretion of T_3 and T_4

c. Hypersecretion of cortisol

d. Hypersecretion of insulin

e. Hyposecretion of T_3 and T_4

f. Hyposecretion of ADH

g. Glucocorticoid and mineralcorticoid deficiency

h. Hyposecretion of insulin

Matching—DKA, HHNC, or Both?

1. _____ Symptoms of hyperglycemia prior to admission

2. _____ History of type 1 diabetes

3. _____ History of type 2 diabetes

4. _____ Flushed, dry skin

5. _____ Acetone breath

6. _____ Develops over time

7. _____ Develops rapidly

8. _____ Kussmaul's respirations

9. _____ Metabolic acidosis

10. _____ Sodium levels elevated

11. _____ Low bicarbonate levels

12. _____ Glucose levels may be > 800 mg/dl

13. _____ More profound dehydration

14. _____ Protein and fat catabolism

15. _____ More common in elderly

a. DKA

b. HHNC

c. Both DKA and HHNC

PERSONALIZE IT!!

❖ This chapter demonstrates the effects of stress on the endocrine system and, ultimately, on health. How much do you think stressful lifestyles influence the incidence of endocrine imbalances? Do you think exercise is an important stress-relief measure? What type of exercise do you do on a regular basis?

❖ Think about your family—do any of your close relatives have diabetes? The incidence of type 2 diabetes is increasing dramatically in the United States, and up to 50% of newly diagnosed diabetics already have complications. This disease is easily diagnosed and often treatable with diet and lifestyle modification. Familiarize yourself with long-term effects of this insidious disease and incorporate patient teaching concerning diabetes in your patient care.

CROSSWORD PUZZLE

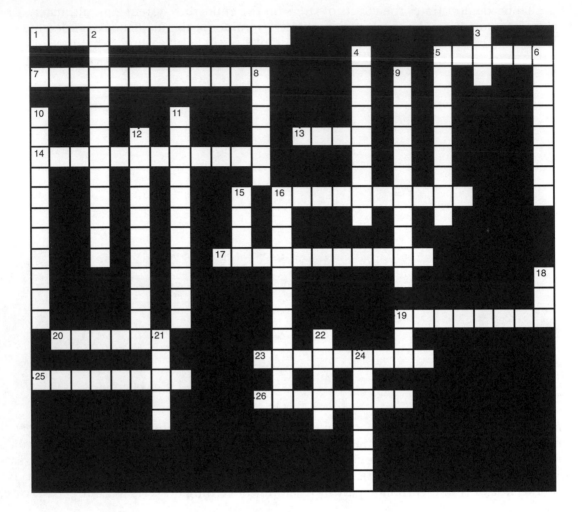

Across

1. Excessive levels of glucose in the blood.
5. SIADH causes a dilution of this electrolyte.
7. High potassium level.
13. Similar to DKA, but with minimal ketosis and no acidosis (abbreviation).
14. Lack of adequate glucose in the blood.
16. Type of diabetes insipidus secondary to neurological problems.
17. Abnormally increased heart rate seen in thyroid storm.
19. Excessive urination seen with diabetes insipidus.
20. Disease associated with hyperthyroidism.
23. Diabetes _____ results from ADH insufficiency.
25. Hormone normally released via stimulation by ACTH.
26. Metabolic _____ is seen in blood gas analysis in DKA.

Down

2. Mg, K^+, and Cl^- are examples of _____.
3. _____ regulates water balance and serum osmolality (abbreviation).
4. Severe stress and _____ can trigger DKA.
5. Drug commonly used for thyroid replacement.
6. _____ coma is extreme hypothyroidism with a hypometabolic state.
8. Assess _____ first in DKA and HHNC.
9. Drug used to treat diabetes insipidus.
10. Problem secondary to DKA and HHNC.
11. Drug given when serum pH is < 7.10.
12. Increases Na^+ reabsorption from the loop of Henle.
15. Type of cells that secrete insulin within the pancreas.
16. Type of diabetes insipidus treated with thiazide diuretic administration.
18. Caused by absolute insulin deficiency (abbreviation).
19. One of two drugs used in the treatment of thyroid storm (abbreviation).
21. Thyroid _____ is extreme hyperthyroidism with serious signs and symptoms.
22. _____ occurs when the body secretes too much ADH (abbreviation).
24. Drug given by infusion to patients with DKA and HHNC.

CONCEPT MAP

You are caring for two patients with diabetic emergencies. Mrs.D. has been diagnosed with DKA; Mrs. H. has HHNC. Fill in expected findings for the following categories for each of your patients.

	Mrs. D (DKA)	Mrs. H (HHNC)
Pathophysiology:		
Health History:		
Clinical Manifestations:		
Diagnostics:		
Patient Education:		

Chapter 16

TRAUMA

LEARNING OUTCOMES

- Describe a systems approach to trauma care.
- Identify mechanisms of traumatic injury commonly seen in the critical care setting.
- Discuss prehospital care, emergency care, and resuscitation of the trauma patient.
- Describe assessment and management of common traumatic injuries.
- Discuss nursing interventions for care of trauma patients, including prevention of complications.

TERMINOLOGY

- blunt versus penetrating trauma
- cavitation
- compartment syndrome
- diagnostic peritoneal lavage (DPL)
- fat embolism
- flail chest
- hemothorax
- kinetic energy
- pericardial tamponade

- pneumothorax
- primary survey
- pulmonary contusion
- rhabdomyolysis
- secondary survey
- tension pneumothorax
- trauma team
- triage
- tri-modal distribution

KEY POINTS

❖ Trauma

- Trauma is injury resulting from an external force; it can be accidental, self-inflicted, or caused by an act of violence. It occurs when an uncontrolled source of energy comes into contact with the body.

  - Kinetic (mechanical), chemical, thermal, electrical, or radiation are types of energy.

  - Trauma is the fourth leading cause of death between the ages of 1 and 44. Over half of traumatic incidents involve drugs, alcohol, or other substance abuse.

  - Trauma is a public health problem; it costs $4 billion health care dollars annually.

- Tri-modal distribution of death due to trauma was introduced in 1982: it refers to three time periods for death due to traumatic injury and is the basis for an organized trauma management system.

  - First peak—seconds to minutes from injury; brain, spinal cord, heart or large vessel lacerations.

  - Second peak—minutes to several hours after injury; hematomas, hemopneumothorax, ruptured spleen, other multiple injuries with significant blood loss.

  - Third peak—several days to weeks after injury; usually sepsis or multiple organ failure (MOF).

- The trauma team is headed by the trauma surgeon; other members have specific preassigned duties.

- The American College of Surgeons Committee on Trauma devised a system of trauma care center levels.

  - Level I—regional resource, state-of-the-art science care, education, outreach, and research; should treat 1200 trauma patients each year.

  - Level II—provides care for trauma patients, transfer to level I if needed, and outreach.

  - Level III—rural hospital with protocols for managing patients and transferring as needed.

  - Level IV—rural clinic with protocols.

- Triage refers to sorting of patients according to specialized care needed. A BP of < 90 mm Hg in an adult trauma victim always requires transport to a trauma center.

- Blunt trauma (more common in rural and suburban areas) is associated with motor vehicle accidents, assault with a blunt object, falls from heights, and sports injuries. Coup and contrecoup and deceleration injuries cause tearing of tissues and vessels. Low-density tissues and structures (lungs) tolerate energy transference well, but high-density solid organs (heart, spleen, liver, kidneys) tolerate it poorly and may rupture.

- Penetrating trauma (more common in inner-city and urban areas) include stab wounds and gunshot or other missile wounds. Foreign objects (glass, wood, clothing) add to injury and risk for infection, but these types of wounds are more easily diagnosed and treated.

- Prehospital treatment involves minimal care with emphasis on ABCs. Care includes establishing an airway, providing ventilation, controlling hemorrhage, stabilizing fractures, establishing IV access and fluid resuscitation, and immobilizing the spine.

- The emergency care phase begins with the primary survey. It is a systematic survey of ABCD: *A*irway patency with cervical immobilization, *B*reathing presence and effectiveness, *C*irculatory status, and *D*isability (overview of neurological condition). Any life-threatening injury is identified and resolved. Baseline vital signs are taken to guide interventions, and continuous pulse oximetry and ECG monitoring are initiated.

- The resuscitation phase involves the secondary survey—a head-to-toe, front-to-back evaluation of actual and potential injury, followed by radiologic and laboratory studies. Data is obtained to establish priorities for care and interventions.

❖ Airway Management

- Many factors can impair the airway: facial fractures and bleeding, vomiting, decreased sensorium, and tongue displacement. Jaw thrust and chin lift maneuvers open the airway without cervical spine impairment. Oral or nasopharyngeal airways can be used if needed in spontaneously breathing patients. Endotracheal intubation is often needed. If unable to intubate, emergency cricothyrotomy is performed.

- Ineffective breathing patterns are caused by a variety of traumatic injuries; ongoing assessment is essential. Supplemental O_2 and ventilatory assistance are provided as needed.

  - Needle thoracostomy is required for treatment of tension pneumothorax; chest tube insertion may follow.

  - Administration of fluids and blood products may be necessary in contusion or hemothorax

- Impaired gas exchange occurs as a result of decrease in inspired air, retained secretions, atelectasis, or hemothorax. Patient may need supplemental oxygen, mechanical ventilation, and restoration of circulating blood volume. Ongoing assessment of oxygen saturation, end-tidal CO_2, and ABGs is needed along with physical assessment.

- Hypovolemic shock occurs as a result of external (hemorrhage) or internal (hemothorax, massive pelvic fractures) causes. Bleeding must first be stopped using pressure or elevation; pneumatic antishock garments (PASG) can be used to apply pressure to abdomen and lower extremities and to stabilize fractures. Some controversy exists about the effectiveness of PASG.

  - Establish two large-bore venous access lines or a central line; isotonic crystalloids such as Ringer's lactate (first choice) and normal saline are given along with blood products based on response to initial fluid resuscitation and lab values. Ongoing assessment of vital signs, urine output, mental status, and hemodynamic parameters are nursing priorities.

  - Three patterns of response are seen:

    - Rapid responders respond quickly and remain hemodynamically stable when infusion is slowed.

    - Transient responders respond initially but deteriorate when infusion slows; indicates continuing loss of blood and need for surgical intervention.

    - Minimal responders need surgical intervention immediately

- Signs of deterioration include falling hematocrit and PaO_2, decreasing urine output, and increased serum lactate levels. CT scan or diagnostic peritoneal lavage may be done to determine source of bleeding.

- Hypothermia (core body temperature < 35° C) is a universal problem with rapid infusion of fluids. It can lead to development of myocardial dysfunction, coagulopathies, reduced perfusion, and impaired metabolism. The triad of hypothermia, acidosis, and coagulopathy is associated with a poor prognosis.

❖ Chest Injuries

- Tension pneumothorax occurs when injury allows air to enter but not escape from the pleural cavity. Increased pressure collapses the lung, then compresses the heart and great vessels toward the unaffected side. This is an emergency and requires immediate decompression using a 14-gauge needle inserted into the second intercostal space, midclavicular line.

- Hemothorax is a collection of blood in the pleural space. Symptoms are decreased breath sounds, dullness to percussion of affected side, hypotension, and respiratory distress. A chest tube is inserted to drain off the blood.

- Open pneumothorax is a sucking wound that allows air to pass in and out of the pleural space. An occlusive dressing is applied, taped on three sides only, until a chest tube can be inserted.

- Cardiac tamponade, generally caused by a penetrating trauma, is a rapid collection of fluid (blood) in the pericardial sac. Classic signs (Beck's triad) are hypotension, muffled heart sounds, and distended neck veins. Pericardiocentesis is performed by needle aspiration.

- Pulmonary contusion is a common cause of death after chest trauma, because of the development of ARDS or pneumonia. Rib fractures or flail chest (three or more adjacent ribs fractured in more than one location, floating freely) often accompany pulmonary contusion. Pain and edematous tissue cause respiratory distress, requiring ventilatory support.

❖ Spinal Cord Injury

- Neurological exam, portable x-rays, and possibly a CT scan are performed after evaluation of ABCs. Postural reduction of a spinal dislocation is done with cervical traction tongs, halo traction devices, or spinal fusion.

  - IV methylprednisolone has been shown to improve outcomes if initiated within 8 hours of injury.

  - Neurogenic shock is common as a result of loss of sympathetic output following cervical spine injury.

❖ Head Injury

- Skull fractures may be linear, basilar, open or closed depressed, or comminuted.

  - Basilar fractures are diagnosed by presence of CSF in the nose or ears, by Battle's sign, hemotympanum, or periorbital ecchymosis.

- Secondary injury refers to complications of the primary injury and includes hypoxemia, hypotension, increased ICP, cerebral edema, hypercapnia, hypothermia, and infection.

❖ Musculoskeletal Injuries

- Fractures can be open or closed and are graded according to degree of bony, soft, vascular and nerve tissue affected. Closed fractures are treated with closed reduction; open fractures with open reduction within 18 hours to prevent infection and nonunion.

- Pelvic fractures are stable or unstable. Unstable pelvic fractures are life-threatening, often have associated hemorrhage, genitourinary tract damage, or sepsis.

- Complications of musculoskeletal injuries include:

  - Compartment syndrome—Localized edema in closed muscle compartments that contain neurovascular bundles. Patients complain of extreme pain unrelieved by narcotics. Distal areas must be assessed for pulse and sensation. Treatment involves elevation of affected limb, removal of external sources of pressure, or surgical fasciotomy.

  - Myoglobinuria results from rhabdomyolysis caused by muscle destruction. When combined with hypovolemia, acute tubular necrosis (ATN) and acute renal failure follow.

  - Fat embolism syndrome can accompany long bone, pelvic, or multiple fractures. Develops 24 to 48 hours after injury. Classic indicators are new-onset tachycardia, low-grade fever, dyspnea, increased respiratory rate and effort, and abnormal ABGs. Intubation and mechanical ventilation (PEEP) may be required. Prevention is the best policy, by stabilizing fractures to minimize bone movement and release of fatty material.

❖ Abdominal Injuries

- The liver is the organ most commonly injured in blunt or penetrating trauma; hemorrhage frequently results. It is diagnosed with diagnostic peritoneal lavage or abdominal CT scan.

- The spleen is most often damaged by blunt trauma. LUQ tenderness, peritoneal irritation, Kehr's sign (referred pain to the left shoulder), hypotension, or signs of hemorrhagic shock are indicators. Loss of the spleen results in impaired immune function, with particular susceptibility to pneumococcal infection. It is also diagnosed by DPL or CT scan.

❖ Critical Care Phase

- A systems approach is used for continuing data collection. Nursing care is focused on maintenance of ABCs and interventions for the specific injury. The most common secondary complications are:

  - ARDS—2 to 48 hours after injury. Acute onset; PaO_2/FiO_2 of 200 mm HG or less; bilateral pulmonary infiltrates; PCWP of 18 mm HG or less; no clinical evidence of left atrial hypertension.

  - Deep vein thrombosis (DVT)—A thrombus generally forms in the lower extremities, breaks free, and becomes lodged in the pulmonary vasculature (pulmonary embolism). Early ambulation, sequential compression devices, and low-dose subcutaneous heparin are preventive measures.

- Risk for infection is high in trauma patients, both from the primary injury and from nosocomial sources. Stressed immune system, poor nutritional status, and exposure to invasive procedures all contribute. Pneumonia is often caused by aspiration at the time of injury. Central venous catheters, especially when placed in the groin, are common sites of infection. Sinusitis can result from nasotracheal or nasogastric tubes.

- Acute renal failure and ATN frequently occur as a result of decreased renal blood flow and increased myoglobin concentration. Decreased urine output is the first indication.

- Multisystem organ failure (MOF) is a syndrome of progressive but potentially reversible organ failure involving two or more organs remote from the primary injury site. Bacterial infection most often leads to MOF. Early identification and treatment are crucial.

- Rehabilitation is essential for all; many trauma victims are young and can return to productive lives with continuing rehabilitation. Early mobilization, nutritional and psychological support, and patient education help minimize complications and maximize rehabilitation potential for all ages.

REVIEW QUESTIONS

True/False

1. **T F**   Traumatic injury is the leading cause of death in the elderly.

2. **T F**   The secondary survey involves obtaining baseline assessment of vital signs.

3. **T F**   Ventilation with 100% oxygen using a bag-valve-mask device should be performed before intubation is attempted.

4. **T F**   Anaerobic metabolism is associated with decreasing serum lactate levels.

5. **T F**   Poor patient prognosis is associated with administration of over 10 units of packed RBCs in a 24-hour period.

6. **T F**   Hyperthermia, acidosis, and coagulopathy during the early treatment phase of trauma victims comprise a triad of high morbidity.

7. **T F**   A suspicion of tension pneumothorax should be confirmed by x-ray before needle thoracotomy is performed.

8. **T F**   Hypotension, muffled heart sounds, and distended neck veins are classic signs of cardiac tamponade.

9. **T F**   Following a cervical spine injury, hypertension and bradycardia are indicative of neurogenic shock.

10. **T F**   Small-volume resuscitation with hypertonic saline solution is the best prehospital intervention for the victim of severe head injury.

Multiple Choice

1. Which of the following is *not* a characteristic of a level 1 trauma care center?

   a. It is a regional resource center.
   b. It conducts major outreach programs for trauma personnel.
   c. Its plan of care includes agreements to transfer patients to acute care centers.
   d. It provides educational programs for trauma personnel.

2. The extent of internal injury is more easily predicted when it results from:

   a. a high-velocity gunshot wound.
   b. a low-velocity gunshot wound.
   c. a stab wound.
   d. shearing forces.

3. A local infection that becomes generalized and causes signs of hypotension and hypoperfusion is referred to as:

   a. bacteremia.
   b. sepsis.
   c. septic shock.
   d. systemic inflammatory response syndrome.

4. As part of the trauma team, you would expect prehospital care of a trauma patient to include all of the following *except*:

   a. cervical spine immobilization and airway management.
   b. large-bore IV access.
   c. crystalloid and blood administration.
   d. splinting of fractures to extremities.

5. Physiological changes you might expect to see in the geriatric population include all of the following *except*:

   a. poor wound healing.
   b. decreased chest wall elasticity.
   c. decreased sensitivity to catecholamines.
   d. decreased myocardial irritability.

6. Your patient was a victim of a motor vehicle accident yesterday and suffered an open fracture of the femur. His condition was stable until an hour ago, when he began to complain of shortness of breath. His heart rate is 104, respiratory rate is 30, BP is 90/60, and temperature is now 38.4° C. You suspect that he:

   a. has developed metabolic acidosis.
   b. is developing SIRS.
   c. has a fat embolism.
   d. is experiencing early MOF.

7. Diagnostic peritoneal lavage can be used to identify intraabdominal bleeding from all of the following organs *except*:

   a. kidney.
   b. small intestine.
   c. spleen.
   d. stomach.

8. In the emergency treatment of _____, the technique of needle thoracostomy is used.

   a. airway obsruction
   b. internal hemorrhage
   c. spinal cord injury
   d. tension pneumothorax

9. Poor patient outcomes are associated with:

 a. chest tube placement for treatment of hemothorax.
 b. immediate decompression of tension pneumothorax.
 c. massive fluid resuscitation.
 d. not fully occluding the dressing on an open pneumothorax dressing.

10. Which of the following is *not* a direct cause of ARDS in trauma patients?

 a. Aspiration of gastric contents
 b. Fat or air embolism
 c. Inhalation injury
 d. Sepsis

PERSONALIZE IT!!

❖ Young people are often victims of motor vehicle accidents and of violence. It seems that TV coverage is dominated by violence and focuses on crime details, rather than on the societal context of these issues. What preventive teaching strategies can you think of to use with families and friends of the victims that you care for?

❖ Urban life in the twenty-first century potentiates many scenarios for disaster. Familiarize yourself with your unit's policies for managing different types of disaster. Do you personally have a plan for child/family/pet care in the event you must remain at work during a disaster?

CROSSWORD PUZZLE

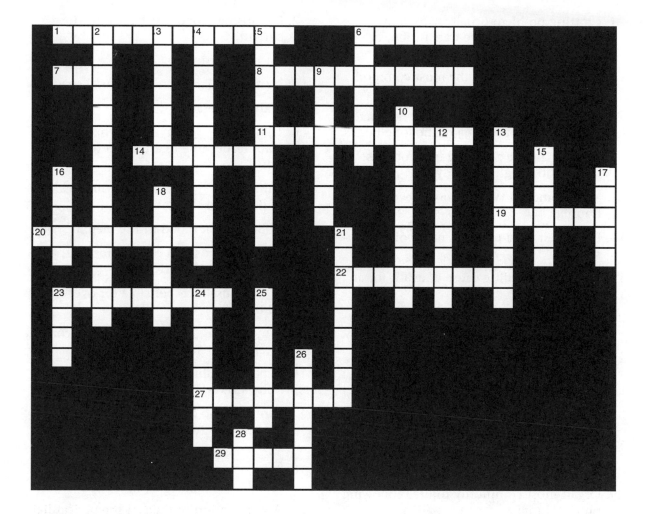

Across

1. Clotting problem usually caused by hypothermia, massive transfusion, or both.

6. Bacterial infection is the most common event leading to this.

7. _____ embolism syndrome is a risk factor associated with trauma of the long bones.

8. Type of trauma resulting from objects impaled through the body.

11. Most common type of shock seen in trauma.

14. Blood test used to assess metabolic acidosis.

19. The fourth leading cause of death for all ages.

20. Most common cause of this condition is aspiration at the time of injury.

22. _____ acidosis results from persistent hypoperfusion.

23. Crush injuries result in release of this substance that can cause acute renal failure.

27. O _____ is the universal donor blood type used in exsanguination.

29. Organ most commonly injured following blunt trauma.

Down

2. Reinfusing blood loss back into the patient.

3. Fat in the urine.

4. Air accumulation in the pleural space.

5. Body temperature < 35° C.

6. Trauma _____; physician who assumes team leader role in a trauma resuscitation.

9. Pulmonary _____ is a fatal complication of deep vein thrombosis.

10. Collection of blood in the pleural space.

12. Open wounds and central lines put the trauma patient at risk for _____.

13. _____ abuse is responsible for over half of all traumas.

15. A method of "sorting" patients according to emergent status.

16. Type of trauma that occurs when the body strikes a stationary object.

17. Term used to describe paradoxical chest movements (the chest rises on expiration).

18. Type of pneumothorax in which air is unable to escape the pleural cavity.

21. Accumulation of fluid in the pericardial sac.

23. Abbreviation for multisystem organ failure.

24. _____ electrolyte solutions most closely resemble the body's natural fluids and are used for initial fluid resuscitation.

25. Type of skull fracture seen clinically with "raccoon eyes."

26. _____ survey is a crucial assessment done in the first 1 to 2 minutes.

28. Type of fracture most commonly seen with chest trauma.

CONCEPT MAP

A 44-year-old construction worker has fallen from a second-story level, landing on a pile of debris. As you assist in transferring him from the stretcher, you notice his chest wall expanding unevenly with respirations. You also observe a sharp piece of metal stuck in his abdomen, and you believe you smell alcohol.

Mechanism of Injury

Primary Survey   **Secondary Survey**

Significant History

Initial Diagnostic Tests   **Anticipated Complications**

Initial Labs

Chapter 17

BURNS

219

KEY POINTS

❖ Incidence

- Burns account for 5500 deaths, 51,000 acute hospital admissions, and 1.25 million total injuries annually, resulting in significant economic and social consequences. Research-based advances in fluid resuscitation, wound care, respiratory and metabolic support, and microbial surveillance have improved survival and recovery.

- High probability of survival exists with burns over less than 81% of the body, but significant morbidity occurs with burns over more than 50% of the body.

- Old and young are at higher risk.

❖ Three Treatment Phases of Burn Care

- Resuscitative (emergent) phase—About 48 hours; most crucial period. Goal is to prevent shock.

- Acute phase—Begins with diuresis; lasts until wound closure (weeks or months). Goal is uncomplicated wound healing and emotional support.

- Rehabilitative phase—Rarely involves the critical care nurse, although the foundation for rehabilitation is laid in the ICU. Goal is to restore functional ability and return to adjusted role and vocation.

❖ The Integumentary System

- Largest organ of the body.

- Epidermis is the outer, thinner, layer.

- Dermis is the inner layer, containing sweat and sebaceous glands, hair follicles, and sensory fibers for pain, pressure, touch, and temperature.

- Subcutaneous tissue is a layer of connective tissue and fat deposits.

- Burn damage to the skin causes loss of body heat, fluids, and regulatory control; loss of protection from infection; loss of sensory input; and loss of cosmetic appearance.

- Depth of injury depends on duration of contact, temperature, amount of tissue exposed, and ability to dissipate heat. Now classified as partial-thickness or full-thickness injury.

  - Partial-thickness injury:

    - Superficial partial-thickness injury may involve epidermis or variable degrees of dermis; heals within 21 days (first- and second-degree burns).

    - Deep partial-thickness injury involves epidermis and most of dermis; heals in 3 to 6 weeks but usually excised and grafted (second-degree burns).

  - Full-thickness injury:

    - Destruction of all layers down to or past subcutaneous fat, fascia, muscle, or bone. Nerves are destroyed, so wound is painless. Always requires grafting (third-degree burn).

  - Three zones of thermal injury:

    - Zone of coagulation—core, greatest area of necrosis

- Zone of stasis—vascular damage and potentially reversible tissue injury

- Zone of hyperemia—minimal injury, similar to superficial partial-thickness injury

❖ Pathophysiology of Burns

- Local response: The heat leads to a pronounced acute inflammatory response. Release of cellular enzymes and vasoactive substances and activation of complement result in increased vessel permeability and fluid shift to extravascular space. Intracellular swelling and leaking of serum proteins obstructs lymph flow.

  - Magnitude of response is proportionate to extent of injury. In extensive burns (over more than 25% of body), edema occurs in both burned and unburned areas.

  - Maximum edema is seen 18 to 24 hours after the burn.

- Systemic response: All organ systems are affected. Hypofunction occurs, then hyperfunction.

  - Cardiovascular—Decreased plasma volume leads to decreased CO, increased SVR, and decreased O_2 delivery. Arterial pressure is maintained by the catecholamine-induced vasoconstrictive response. Blood flow is redistributed to perfuse essential viscera. With adequate fluid resuscitation, CO is normalized in 24 hours and remains supranormal until wound closure.

  - Host defense mechanisms—Immune defects are not clearly understood. End result is overstimulation of suppressor T cells, activation of complement, and depression of helper T, killer T, and polymorphonuclear leukocyte activity. Risk for sepsis is high.

  - Pulmonary—Initial transient pulmonary hypertension. Smoke inhalation brings increased risk of mortality. Inhalation injury is classified as (1) from carbon monoxide, (2) above the glottis, and (3) below the glottis.

  - Renal—Biphasic response of initial oliguria due to decreased plasma flow and GFR, followed by (sometimes modest) diuresis secondary to increased CO.

  - GI—Ileus may occur secondary to hypovolemia and neurological and endocrine responses. Antacids and/or H_2 histamine blockers are needed to protect gastric mucosal.

  - Metabolic—Hypermetabolism follows fluid resuscitation, possibly because of catecholamine secretion. Peak hypermetabolic rates reached at 6 to 10 days postburn.

- Thermal injury: 90% of injuries, skin contact with heat source. Severity proportionate to degree and duration of exposure.

  - Exposure to 60° C (hot water heater temperature) causes tissue destruction in 3 to 5 seconds.

  - Children and elderly are more susceptible.

- Chemical injury: 10% of injuries. Severity related to type, volume, and concentration of agent and duration of contact. Damage continues until the agent is completely removed.

  - Alkalis (cleaning products)—Produce liquefaction necrosis. Cause more damage than acids.

  - Acids (bathroom cleaners, rust removers, swimming pool chemicals)—Cause coagulation necrosis and precipitation of protein.

- Organic compounds (phenols and petroleum products)—Cause chemical burns and systemic effects. Coagulation necrosis, CNS depression, hypothermia, hypotension, pulmonary edema, and intravascular hemolysis can result from phenols. Gasoline can cause skin necrosis, pneumonitis and bronchitis, and hepatic and renal damage.

- Electrical injury: High voltage (> 1000 volts) or low voltage (< 1000 volts). Tissue damage results from conversion of electrical energy into heat. Both alternating and direct current are dangerous, but AC is more likely to cause cardiac arrest and has tetanic effect (locks victim to source of electricity). Superficial tissues cool faster; deep tissue necrosis can occur below viable tissue. Monitor for cardiac dysrhythmias.

  - Lightning often produces superficial cutaneous injury but may cause cardiopulmonary arrest and transient but severe CNS deficits.

- Toxic epidermal necrolysis syndrome (TENS) or Stevens-Johnson's syndrome (SJS): Rare condition of exfoliative dermatitis in response to some agent—most commonly a drug reaction (sulfa, phenobarbitol, or phenytoin). High mortality due to immune suppression complications such as sepsis and pneumonia. Painful partial-thickness injury occurs.

- Staphylococcal scalded skin (SSS) or Ritter's disease: More common in children; a reaction to staphylococcal toxin. Similar to TENS but with low mortality; treated with antibiotic therapy.

Assessment	Resuscitative Phase	Acute Care Phase
Respiratory	Assess breath sounds; work of breathing; sputum color and consistency; symmetry of chest excursion. Monitor for O_2 saturation; impaired gas exchange (carbon monoxide or inhalation); ineffective airway clearance (tracheal edema).	Continue to monitor for signs of respiratory compromise and potential pneumonia. May see tachypnea, abnormal breath sounds, purulent secretions.
Cardiovascular	Assess fluid volume r/t capillary permeability; VS; urine output; baseline weight; cardiac rhythm; electrolytes. Check peripheral pulses. PA catheter is useful in major burns with inhalation injury.	Monitor for complications r/t fluid resuscitation. Monitor daily weight, I&O, frequent VS. Monitor PA catheter if present.
Neurological	Initially awake, alert, oriented. Watch for changes in LOC (r/t hypoxemia and/or hypovolemia).	LOC changes reflect hypoxemia, hypoperfusion, or sepsis.
Renal	Monitor urine volume, color, and concentration. Oliguria = inadequate fluid resuscitation.	Monitor I&O. Moderate diuresis. Glycosuria is early sign of sepsis if patient is not diabetic.
GI	Assess bowel sounds, abdominal distention, bleeding, gastric pH, gastric contents. Possible stress response = ulcer development.	Monitor daily calorie counts. Monitor for stress ulcer formation.

Assessment	Resuscitative Phase	Acute Care Phase
Integumentary	Asses depth and extent; edema. High risk for infection.	Assess healing, depth conversion, signs of infection. Monitor temperature closely. Hypothermia from heat loss from open wounds.
Psychosocial	High risk for anxiety in patient and family. Assess early for rehabilitation planning.	Burns are a lifelong injury. Focus on coping ability; look for regression or depression.
Blood, fluid, electrolytes		Hyponatremia, if present, usually resolves in 1 week. Hypernatremia is usually due to evaporation losses. Hypokalemia, hypoproteinemia, negative nitrogen balance, metabolic acidosis may occur. Leukopenia may occur r/t silver sulfadiazine.

Nursing Diagnoses (see text for full explanation)

Resuscitative Phase	Acute Care Phase
• Ineffective airway clearance • Impaired gas exchange • Fluid volume deficit • Altered tissue perfusion • Risk for infection • Altered tissue perfusion: bowel (ileus) • Hypothermia • Acute pain • Risk for injury: GI stress response • Ineffective coping • Impaired skin integrity	• Fluid volume deficit • Impaired skin integrity • Altered nutrition (less than required) • Impaired physical mobility/self-care deficit • Altered family processes • Knowledge deficit: discharge goals • Risk for impaired gas exchange r/t prolonged ventilatory support

❖ Prehospital Intervention

- Early care has a positive impact on recovery.
- First priority is to stop the burning process and prevent further injury.
- Primary survey:
  - ABCs and cervical spine assessment.
  - O_2 therapy if smoke inhalation is suspected
- Secondary survey:
  - Rapid head-to-toe assessment to rule out additional trauma.
  - Victim is usually alert. Obtain history, source of burns, allergies, medical problems, medications, history of tetanus immunization, and current weight.

- Prior to transport, patient is covered with a clean, dry sheet to prevent further contamination and hypothermia. IV access is established in non-burned tissue. Morphine sulfate is the drug of choice for pain.

❖ Resuscitative Phase (ER)

- ABCs reassessed; intubation if needed. Assess for full-thickness circumferential burns of the thorax or extremities; immediate chest wall or peripheral escharotomy may be needed. Fasciotomy may be needed for deep electrical burns.

- Chest x-ray, cervical x-ray (if appropriate), and ECG done on admission.

- Nasogastric tube is generally placed because of frequent development of ileus.

- No intramuscular injections are given because of poor perfusion of edematous tissue.

- ALL jewelry and constrictive clothing must be removed (and secured) to prevent further injury as edema develops.

- Initial estimate of injury with the rule of nines, in which the surface area of various anatomic parts represents 9% of the total body surface area (TBSA); varies with adult/child.

- Fluid resuscitation needs are estimated by body weight, percentage of burn area, and age; first half is given in the first 8 hours, second half over the next 16 hours. Volume is titrated to ensure adequate urine output.

  - For example: 3 ml LR/kg/% of burn. Patient weighs 60 kg and has a 50% burn. 3 x 60 x 50 = 9000 ml; 4500 ml given in first 8 hours, 2250 ml each for next two 8-hour periods.

  - Children require relatively more fluid because of greater TBSA-to-mass ratio.

  - High-voltage burns require more fluid resuscitation in order to flush out accumulation of myoglobin because of hemochromogen release from deep tissue damage.

❖ Transfer to Burn Center

- American Burn Association has guidelines for determining appropriateness of transfer to a burn center. Transfer occurs early in the postburn period.

  - More than 5% TBSA of full-thickness injury.

  - Partial- and full-thickness injury of 10% TBSA in patients under 10 years or over 50 years of age; 20% TBSA in all other ages.

  - Burns of face, hands, feet, genitalia, perineum, or major joints; electrical or chemical burns; inhalation burns; preexisting chronic disease; associated trauma.

- Acute care phase interventions:

  - Monitor critical indices every hour, including peripheral pulses and urine output. Check urine specific gravity, glucose and ketone levels, gastric pH, and occult blood tests every 2 hours. Monitor daily weights.

  - Edema management—Elevate head of bed. Perform range-of-motion exercises for 5 minutes every hour. Monitor titration of fluid resuscitation. Do hourly neurological checks.

  - Pulmonary artery pressure—Monitor if cardiovascular disease is present.

- Electrolyte levels—Monitor according to patient status. Check ABGs, daily chest x-ray for extensive burns or inhalation.

- Hypothermia must be avoided, since wound therapy and skin loss potentiate heat loss.

- Bowel sounds are assessed frequently; early enteral or oral feedings are necessary for healing.

- Pain control—Monitor resting pain, procedural pain, and breakthrough pain. There is usually a mixture of burn depths, so at least part of the wound is sensate. Pain medication should be given prior to debridement, hydrotherapy, surgical intervention, and dressing changes. Opiates are generally used (morphine). PCA is effective because it gives patients a sense of control over their pain.

  - Explanation of procedures and use of imagery and relaxation techniques are helpful.

  - Anxiolytics and benzodiazepines are often used.

- Infection control—Aseptic management of wound and environment; knowledgeable use of topical antibacterial agents; careful use of systemic antibiotics; nutritional support.

❖ Wound management goals are removal of nonviable tissue to promote re-epithelialization and prompt coverage with skin grafts when necessary. Wounds are cleansed with mild soap or surgical disinfectant, rinsed with warm water, then treated in either the open or occlusive method.

- Open method—Burns are left open to air after antimicrobial agent is applied.

- Occlusive method—Wound is covered with gauze saturated with a topical antimicrobial agent (or gauze is placed over treated skin). Net bandages hold the dressings in place.

- A partial- or full-thickness wound that requires more than two weeks for healing, or involves the face, hands, feet, or a joint is treated with autograft skin application. Faster healing with less scar formation and shorter hospitalization are achieved.

  - Split-thickness sheet skin graft may be used intact or may be expanded in a mesh dermatome; full-thickness grafts are used for deeper burns.

  - Special protocols guide the care of the donor and graft sites.

  - Biologic or biosynthetic dressings are often used as temporary coverings for freshly excised wounds until autograft skin is available.

❖ Areas of Special Concern

- Facial burns: May signal inhalation injury. Edema may compromise airway. Good oral hygiene and daily hair removal are necessary.

- Ears: Prone to inflammation and infection (chondritis). Special foam donut is used to prevent pressure.

- Eyes: Frequent application of artificial tears protects cornea and conjunctiva from drying. Eyelashes may invert and scratch cornea.

- Hands or feet: Range-of-motion exercises prevent muscle atrophy. Splinting may be needed to prevent deformity.

- Genitalia and perineum: Meticulous wound care is necessary because of high risk for fecal contamination. Indwelling urethral catheter is often needed.

- Nutrition: Major burns produce a stress-induced hypermetabolic-catabolic response. Sufficient calorie intake and additional nitrogen intake are individualized to ensure a positive nitrogen balance. Tube feedings started in first 24 hours promote positive outcomes.

- Psychosocial: The devastating sequelae of a burn injury require a great deal of emotional support. Psychological adaptation occurs in stages—survival anxiety, search for meaning, investment in recuperation, investment in rehabilitation, and reintegration of identity.

- Geriatric considerations: Fluid resuscitation is challenging in the presence of pre-existing cardiovascular or pulmonary disease. Wound healing is slower because of thinning of skin and poor nutritional status. Complications of immobility have a greater impact on the elderly.

- Prevention is the best strategy!

REVIEW QUESTIONS

Multiple Choice

1. Guidelines for burn center referral call for transfer of a patient with what percentage of total body surface area of full-thickness injury?

   a. 5%
   b. 10%
   c. 15%
   d. 20%

2. The most crucial phase of treatment in burn care is the:

   a. acute phase.
   b. dysfunctional phase.
   c. rehabilitative phase.
   d. resuscitation phase.

3. A major complication of electrical burn injury is acute renal failure caused by:

   a. direct effects of current.
   b. excess fluid resuscitation.
   c. high urine concentration of hemochromagen.
   d. muscle destruction.

4. The rule of nines is used as an assessment tool and must be adjusted according to what variation in children?

   a. Extremity size
   b. Proportion of back size
   c. Proportion of head size
   d. No adjustment needed

5. What zone of thermal injury is the site of minimal cell involvement?

   a. Coagulation
   b. Hyperemia
   c. Hyperstasis
   d. Stasis

6. Applying ice to a burn injury:

   a. is a comfort measure for the patient.
   b. is never recommended because vasoconstriction and hypothermia cause further damage.
   c. prevents further injury in electrical burns.
   d. prevents nerve damage in partial-thickness burns.

7. The first priority in prehospital treatment is to stop the burning. Continuing care of a patient with a chemical burn includes:

   a. applying loose gauze dressings.
   b. cooling the area.
   c. determining the time of the last meal.
   d. removal of the clothing.

8. Mrs. Aloe has sustained second- and third-degree burns over 60% of TBSA. Shortly after admission, her BP drops rapidly. You know this is primarily due to:

   a. extreme pain.
   b. hypovolemic shock.
   c. internal hemorrhage.
   d. psychogenic shock.

9. Your patient weighs 60 kg and has a 40% TBSA burn injury. Fluid resuscitation orders are for 4 ml/kg lactated Ringer's solution. What volume will be infused during the first 8 hours?

   a. 2400 ml
   b. 3600 ml
   c. 4800 ml
   d. 9600 ml

10. Burn wounds tend to heal in positions of nonfunction and:

    a. abduction.
    b. contraction.
    c. extension.
    d. opposition.

11. Silver nitrate is a topical medication used in burn wound care because it:

    a. functions as a dermal layer to the skin.
    b. is effective against most gram-positive and gram-negative wound pathogens.
    c. is effective against a wide spectrum of wound pathogens and fungal infections.
    d. is used as a temporary wound cover.

Matching—Burn Wound Care

1. _____ Alloderm®

2. _____ Allograft (homograft) skin

3. _____ Biobrane®

4. _____ Biological dressing

5. _____ Biosynthetic dressing

6. _____ Integra® ("artificial skin")

7. _____ Transcyte®

8. _____ Xenograft (heterograft) skin

a. Wound covering composed of both biological and synthetic materials.

b. Temporary wound cover of human or animal species tissue.

c. Temporary wound covering made up of a collagen base of human neonatal fibroblasts injected into a matrix.

d. Dermal replacement allowing use of a thin epithelial autograft; transplantable tissue consisting of human cryopreserved allogenic dermis from which the epidermal, fibroblast, and endothelial cells targeted for immune response have been removed.

e. Two-layer wound dressing: a "dermal" layer made of animal collagen that interfaces with an open wound surface, and an "epidermal" layer made of Silastic that controls water loss and acts as a bacterial barrier. The dermal layer biodegrades within several months and is resorbed. The epidermal layer may be removed and replaced with autograft skin when appropriate.

f. Temporary wound cover composed of a graft of skin transplanted from another human, living or dead.

g. Bilaminate wound dressing composed of nylon mesh enclosed in a collagen derivative with a silicon rubber outer membrane; permeable to some antibiotic ointments.

h. Temporary wound cover to promote healing. A graft (usually pigskin) is transplanted between animals of different species.

PERSONALIZE IT!!

❖ Older adults are more prone to burn injuries because of diminished manual dexterity, reaction time, visual acuity, hearing, and judgment. What preventive teaching can you do for your own grandparents, parents, and elderly neighbors?

❖ Many home water heaters are set at 60° C (140° F). Exposure to this temperature can cause tissue damage in as little as 3 to 5 seconds. Young children are especially prone to scald injuries. A valuable patient teaching tip is advising families with young children or elderly to decrease their water temperature. Do you know how to adjust the thermostat on a water heater?

CROSSWORD PUZZLE

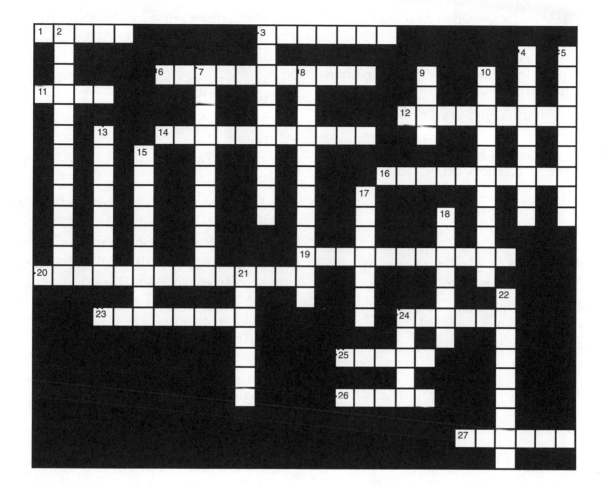

Across

1. A skin _____ is needed to treat full-thickness burns.

3. _____-thickness injury involves burns through the epidermis or variable portion of the dermis.

6. Incision through burned tissue to restore circulation.

11. _____-thickness burns are major burns through epidermis, dermis, and possibly bone.

12. Changes in appearance associated with burns may result in a disturbance of _____ (2 words).

14. Burn patients must be kept warm to prevent this complication.

16. Breakdown of protein stores seen in burn victims.

19. Route for giving pain medication to the burn victim.

20. Important aspect of burn care.

23. Patients with inhalation injuries must be assessed for carbon _____.

24. _____ must be assessed, especially in victims of smoke inhalation.

25. Common GI alteration in resuscitative phase.

26. The rule of _____ is used to rapidly estimate the total body percentage burned.

27. Minimum desired urine output is _____ ml/hour.

Down

2. Most crucial phase for the burn patient.

3. _____ pulses should be assessed for circulatory function.

4. Watch for too much of this electrolyte in burn patients.

5. The zone of _____ is an area of minimal injury.

7. This syndrome results in occlusion of circulation.

8. Term used when fluid accumulates in the interstitial space (2 words).

9. If _____ is assessed in the nose or mouth, anticipate respiratory complications.

10. Best assessment of fluid-volume status in the burn patient (2 words).

13. Renal problem seen in resuscitative phase.

15. Alterations in skin integrity make the burn patient especially susceptible to this complication.

17. To remove dead tissue.

18. Example of a first-degree burn.

21. Type of injury caused by exposure to heat.

22. Substance released from damaged tissue that may cause renal failure.

24. Phase that lasts until wound closure.

CONCEPT MAP

Mr. Elmo, 83, accidentally set fire to himself when he lit a cigarette after spilling lighter fluid down the front of his shirt. His burns cover 25% TBSA and are mostly on his abdomen, forehead, and right hand. Mr. Elmo weighs 65 kg.

LOCAL RESPONSE
Cellular injury due to heat

Altered vascular membrane permeability

Fluid resuscitation required:

SYSTEMIC RESPONSE

Skin	Cardio-vascular	Host Defense Mechanism	Pulmonary	Renal	GI	Metabolic
			Inhalation Injury			

ANSWER KEY

CHAPTER 1

True/False

1. F   Critical care nursing deals with patients and families and teaches prevention as well as cure.

Multiple Choice

1. d   Critical care nurses practice in emergency rooms, stepdown units, and long-term care facilities, as well as in intensive care units.
2. d   All are important forms of advocacy.
3. a   The nurse interacts with others as an equal.
4. a   Both criteria must be met.

CHAPTER 2

True/False

1. T
2. F   Nonpharmacologic interventions such as backrubs, dimming lights at night, and clustering nursing activities are preferable.
3. T
4. F   Urine volume peaks from late morning to early afternoon.
5. F   Peer praise is very effective in preventing burnout.

Multiple Choice

1. c   An already confused patient may think you are talking about him or her.
2. c   Psychological stressors often have physical manifestations.
3. b   Researchers have been unable to explain this phenomenon, but postcardiac surgery patients are more apt to suffer from ICU syndrome.
4. d   Nurses must understand that this anger is not really directed at them, but rather results from feelings of helplessness.

5. b Families appreciate timely, understandable information given in a compassionate manner.
6. a Business executives are accustomed to being in control; it is difficult for them to feel dependent on others.

CHAPTER 3

True/False

1. T
2. F The fact that there are *not* reliable methods for determining the extent of brain damage creates many difficult situations.
3. T
4. F There is no absolute list of criteria for determining brain death.

Multiple Choice

1. b It is legally as well as ethically wrong to go against the expressed wishes of a patient as written in a DNR order.
2. c Duty owed, duty breached, injury to patient, and injury due to breach are criteria for malpractice.
3. d Beneficence, nonmaleficence, and justice are represented here.
4. a An ethics committee should be interdisciplinary and should focus on issues of concern to all.
5. d The other three answers are considered extraordinary care.
6. d Comfort measures are continued for all patients regardless of resuscitation status.
7. b Principles of justice and respect for the person dictate that social and economic status are not factors relevant to nursing care.

Matching—Ethical Principles

1. d
2. b
3. f
4. a
5. e
6. c
7. g

CHAPTER 4

Multiple Choice

1. d Automaticity, contractility, and conductivity are all characteristics of cardiac cells. Myomaticity is not a real word.
2. c Dysrhythmia can be caused by defects in impulse formation (as in irritability) or conduction (as in AV delay).

3. d Depolarization normally begins in the SA node and is conducted through the internodal pathways to the AV node, which delays conduction briefly for ventricular filling; it then moves down the bundle of His, which divides into right and left bundle branches; finally it moves deep into the ventricles by way of the Purkinje fibers.
4. b Using the rule of 1500, 1500/20 = 75.
5. a The T wave immediately follows the QRS complex and represents ventricular repolarization. Hyperkalemia often causes tall peaked T waves.
6. d Potassium plays an important role in the depolarization/repolarization process. Low levels facilitate the development of ventricular dysrhythmias.
7. b Coughing, gagging, vomiting, or the Valsalva maneuver temporarily suppresses conduction and therefore heart rate.
8. c Contraction of the atria sends approximately 30% more blood to the ventricles.
9. b Digitalis in toxic doses can be stimulating to the myocardium, especially the atria.
10. a "F" waves of a flutter pattern arise from a single irritable focus in the atrium.
11. d All choices are true. MAT is the same as WAP but faster and with more pronounced hemodynamic effects—primarily lower CO and BP.
12. a Antidysrhythmics act in different ways and are not free of side effects. They are effective for both atrial and ventricular dysrhythmias.
13. b Atrial flutter is characterized by a sawtooth pattern, an atrial rate of 250–350 beats per minute, an often irregular ventricular rhythm with conduction of every second, third, or fourth beat.
14. d Ventricular tachycardia is present when more than 3 PVCs occur in a row at a rate of 130–250 beats per minute. No P waves are seen; QRS complexes are consistent in appearance.
15. a Atrial fibrillation is characterized by a wavy baseline, no detectable P waves, and an irregularly irregular ventricular rhythm.
16. a Atrial fibrillation is described in answer 15. The PVCs are similar in appearance, indicating that they are originating from one area, or are unifocal.

Fill In the Blanks

a. < 0.11 second
b. 0.12–0.20 second
c. 0.06–0.10 second

Matching—Precordial Leads

1. c
2. b
3. d
4. f
5. a
6. e

Matching—Wave Interpretation

1. c
2. e
3. d
4. g
5. h
6. b
7. a
8. f

Chapter 4 Crossword

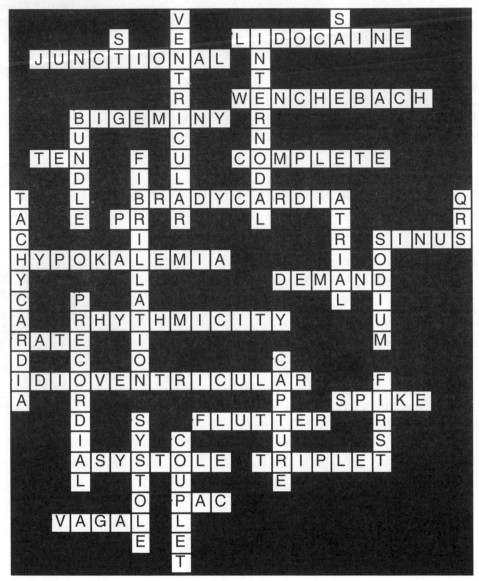

CHAPTER 5

True/False

1. F Cardiac output is the amount of blood ejected from the heart per minute. It is equal to the heart rate x stroke volume.
2. F The phlebostatic axis is located at the fourth intercostal space, midclavicular line.
3. F The AACN found that heparin significantly affects the patency of arterial pressure lines.
4. F MAP closely estimates the perfusion pressure in the aorta and its major branches.
5. T

Multiple Choice

1. c This explanation is understandable for the patient, as well as accurate.

2. d Measurements taken in side-lying positions are significantly different; supine and flat or with head of bed slightly elevated is the standard.

3. a Trendelenburg position promotes venous filling in the upper body, for easier catheter insertion and prevention of air embolism.

4. c

5. a The first CO may be erroneous, especially if the catheter is filled with room-temperature fluid and iced injectate is used. An average of three measurements is more accurate.

6. d Blood returns to the PA from various organs that have different oxygen needs. The blood is mixed in the PA and therefore reflects an overall picture.

7. b Infection is a serious risk imposed by any invasive procedure.

Matching—Key Terms and Concepts

1. l
2. a
3. f
4. j
5. m
6. h
7. d
8. k
9. b
10. i
11. c
12. g
13. e

Chapter 5 Crossword

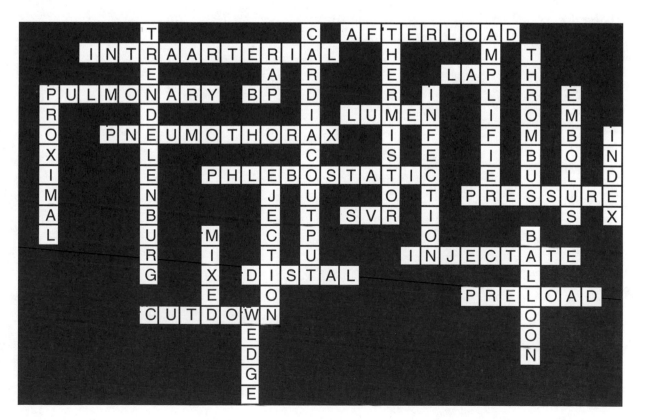

CHAPTER 6

True/False

1. F   There are many potential complications of mechanical ventilation: barotrauma, acid-base disturbances, aspiration, infection, and dependence.
2. F   In hyperventilation, CO_2 (acid) is blown off, resulting in respiratory alkalosis.
3. T
4. T
5. F   Suctioning should be performed only as needed to minimize risk for infection.
6. F   Recent studies do not support routine instillation of saline for suctioning. Patient hydration and use of aerosolized mucolytics are safer and more effective.

Multiple Choice

1. b   Compliance is a measure of the force required to distend the lungs; damage from emphysema increases compliance.
2. b   Elevated levels of carbon dioxide provide the stimulus to breathe in a normal person. In a patient with COPD, the stimulus may be hypoxia instead since CO_2 levels are chronically elevated.
3. c   Retained CO_2 acts as an acid; therefore, respiratory acidosis occurs with inadequate ventilation.
4. a   The first action by the nurse is to check all connections and assess the patient.
5. c   Weaning a patient from the ventilator is a process that must be individualized.
6. d O_2 is in the normal range; the alkalotic pH has not been compensated.

Matching—Key Terms

1. c
2. h
3. f
4. g
5. d
6. b
7. a
8. e

Chapter 6 Crossword

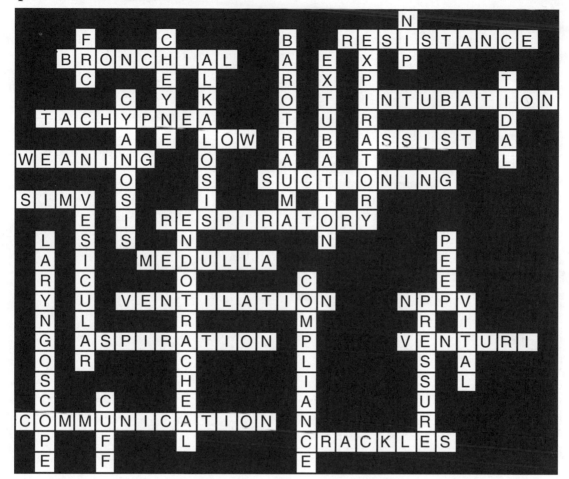

CHAPTER 7

True/False

1. T
2. F Improper head position is the most common cause of inability to ventilate a patient.
3. F Adult chest compressions should depress the sternum by 1.5 to 2 inches.
4. T
5. F Chest pain is less frequently the main symptom of acute MI in the elderly population.
6. T
7. F The crash cart and defibrillator are checked every 24 hours.
8. F Lethal dysrhythmias are V fib/V tach, asystole, and PEA. Note also that symptomatic bradycardias and tachycardias may lead to cardiopulmonary arrest and also must be treated.
9. F Classic bradycardia is a HR < 60 BPM. The broader definition includes symptomatic bradycardia of any type.
10. T

Multiple Choice

1. c   Code activation and CPR are the first priorities.
2. b   Early defibrillation increases the chance of survival. Drug therapy is added as necessary.
3. a   These medications can be diluted in NS and administered via the ETT.
4. b   Ventilation of the intubated patient should not be synchronized to chest compressions.
5. d   Assess the patient—HR is within normal limits; then perform 12-lead ECG for rhythm diagnosis.
6. a   Respiratory acidosis results from buildup of excess CO_2 and metabolic acidosis from anaerobic metabolism.
7. b   Adenosine is the initial drug of choice for SVT, which is narrow-complex. It slows conduction through the AV node and interrupts reentrant conduction.
8. b   Drugs such as epinephrine stimulate beta-adrenergic receptors, increasing heart rate and contractility, thus increasing CO.
9. b   Dopamine's effects are dose-related. At low doses, renal perfusion is increased.
10. d   Nitrates are potent vasodilators, causing flushing and headache, which are dose-related.

Matching—Pharmacology

1. i
2. d
3. l
4. j
5. m
6. e
7. g
8. k
9. o
10. p
11. n
12. c
13. q
14. f
15. h

Chapter 7 Crossword

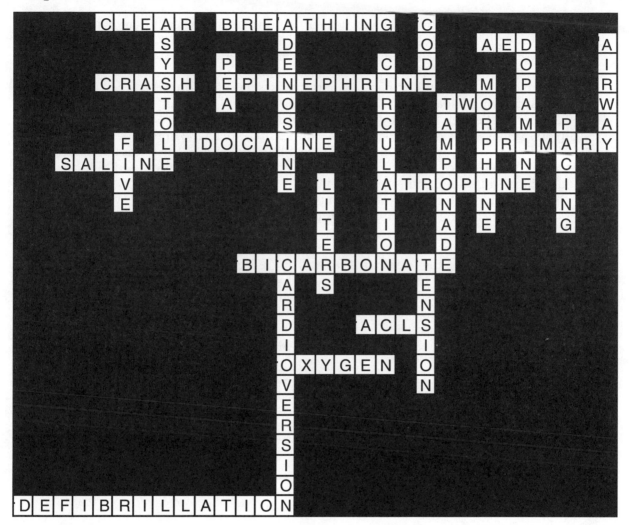

CHAPTER 8

True/False

1. F The cells undergo anaerobic metabolism.
2. F The best position is one in which the lower extremities are elevated slightly.
3. T
4. F SIRS is the initial stage of progressive deterioration in septic shock.
5. F Transient responders respond to the initial bolus but deteriorate as fluids are slowed to a maintenance level, indicating ongoing blood loss or inadequate resuscitation.
6. T
7. T
8. F Packed RBCs increase the blood volume and oxygen carrying capacity without causing the problems of fluid overload associated with the administration of whole blood.
9. F Positive inotropic agents such as dopamine are used to increase the contractile force of the heart in the management of cardiogenic and distributive shock. Fluids are given in hypovolemic shock.
10. T

Multiple Choice

1. c   Microcirculatory functions include delivering nutrients to the cells, removing waste from the cells, and regulating blood volume.
2. c   Cardiogenic shock occurs when diseased coronary arteries are not capable of meeting the O_2 demand of working myocardial cells, resulting in AMI.
3. b   Disturbance in sympathetic nerve impulses causes vasodilation, which decreases SVR, venous return, preload, and CO.
4. c   Vascular dilation in distributive shock increases vascular capacity, creating a relative hypovolemia, decreased venous return, and resultant decreased preload.
5. b   The antigen-antibody reaction causes cellular breakdown and the release of powerful vasoactive substances from the cells, which cause vasodilation, increased capillary permeability, and smooth muscle contraction.
6. a   Decreased BP is detected by carotid sinus and aortic receptors, causing sympathetic stimulation. Epinehprine and norepinephrine are released in an attempt to maintain tissue perfusion.
7. b   Renin is released from the JG cells and reacts with angiotensin to produce angiotensin I. Renin also activates the release of ADH and aldosterone.
8. d   Prolonged inadequate tissue perfusion contributes to MOF.
9. b   The CNS is the most sensitive to changes in the supply of O_2 and nutrients.
10. b   Because peripheral circulation is decreased, pulse oximetry may be inaccurate; ABGs may be required.

Matching—Key Terms

1. j
2. g
3. e
4. b
5. h
6. a
7. c
8. i
9. d
10. f

Chapter 8 Crossword

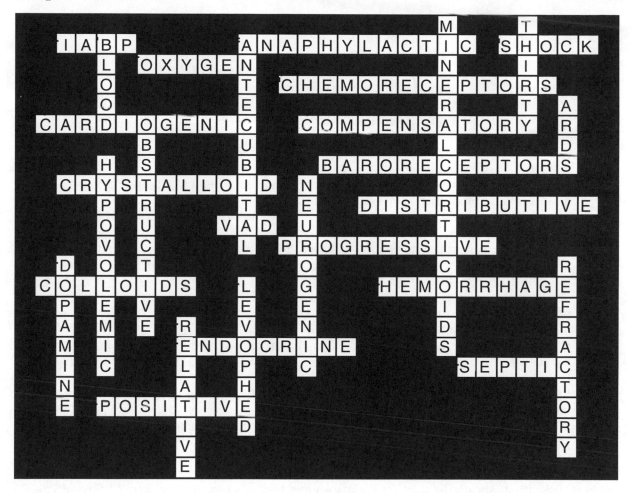

CHAPTER 9

True/False

1. T
2. F Treatment measures for AMI are aimed at reducing the myocardial workload.
3. T
4. F Coronary artery dissection is the most common major complication of PTCA. Hypotension is a minor complication.
5. T
6. F If a pacemaker fails to capture, the electrical stimulus is not depolarizing the myocardium; no QRS will be seen.
7. F The therapeutic range for digoxin is very small; digitalis toxicity is common.
8. F Range of motion is avoided initially to prevent the pacing catheter from dislodging.
9. F Hypotension is a major side effect of nitrate therapy that must be closely monitored.
10. T

Multiple Choice

1. d Major coronary arteries are the RCA and the two branches of the LCA—the LAD and left circumflex

2. b The left circumflex supplies posterior left ventricle and left atrium

3. d A galloping heartbeat is heard with the bell of the stethoscope and is a sign of a severely failing heart.

4. c ECG identifies a baseline rhythm. Radioisotopes show abnormal myocardial cells. Catheterization measures pressures within heart chambers. Echocardiogram is an acoustic imaging procedure and does all of these things.

5. d Both troponins and CK-MB are cardiac-specific and show changes within hours of a myocardial infarct.

6. d The nurse needs to assess, observe, and report type and degree of pain and the effects of NTG. O_2 therapy decreases cell damage.

7. d These are the criteria that distinguish unstable angina from stable and variant (Prinzmetal's) types.

8. a Negative pressure is the normal state. Lung, not pleural space, is reexpanded.

9. a Bumetanide is given as a diuretic, aminophylline is given to assist in gas exchange, and morphine is given to increase venous capacitance.

10. b Cardiotonics (digitalis preparations) are given to CHF patients to improve cardiac output. The nurse must observe for S&S of digitalis toxicity, especially if patients were taking this medication previously.

11. d Dysrhythmias are common after an MI; a change in LOC would be an indicator of possible stroke or hemodynamic fluctuation, and oozing from the IV site must be addressed.

12. a In right-sided failure, blood backs up in the vena cava and systemic circulation, distending visceral veins, especially the hepatic vein. The liver and spleen become engorged, and extremities become edematous.

13. c Filling of the enlarged ventricle causes a vibration during diastole, heard as a gallop.

14. b Cardiac arteriography demonstrates specific areas of partial or complete occlusion. Saphenous vein angiography is not generally performed.

15. d Chest pain that lasts longer than 30 minutes is indicative of an AMI.

16. a The patient should be kept on bedrest in low Fowler's position for 6 to 8 hours after a PTCA. Fluids remove dye from the system, heparin decreases the risk of arterial reocclusion, and chest pain is treated.

Chapter 9 Crossword

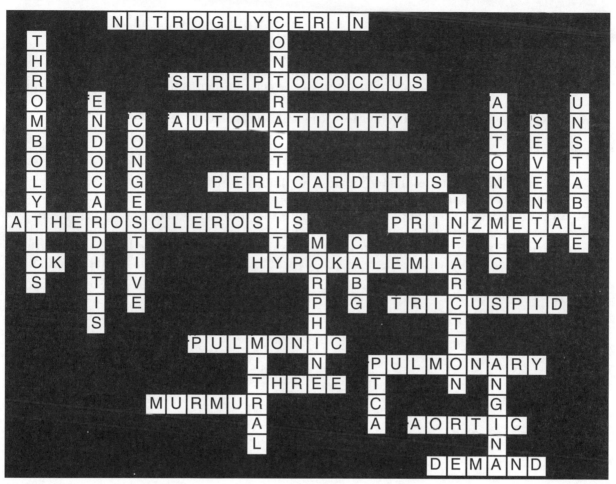

CHAPTER 10

True/False

1. F This describes the basal ganglia. The thalamus acts as the sensory relay.
2. T
3. F Coma develops at < 20 mg/100 ml. Confusion develops at < 70 mg/100 ml.
4. F The pons does this. The hypothalamus controls temperature, water balance, appetite and thirst, cardiovascular regulation, and pituitary hormones.
5. F The brachial plexus innervates the arms. The neck and shoulders are innervated by the cervical plexus (C1–C4).
6. T
7. F This describes cerebellar tonsillar herniation.
8. T
9. T
10. T

Multiple Choice

1. c Hypertension increases CBF and hypotension causes ischemia.

2. b *Sub* means "below" or "beneath." The pia mater lies beneath the subarachnoid membrane.
3. c Babinski's reflex is the classic indicator for neuropathology in the adult.
4. a If stimulation is stopped, this moderately high reading may return to normal.
5. a LOC is the earliest and most direct reflection of neurological status.
6. c Violent seizures put the patient a greatest risk for head injury.
7. a Central herniation is a downward shift of the cerebral hemispheres, basal ganglia, and diencephalon through the tentorial notch.
8. b CN III, IV, and VI work together for extraocular movements.
9. b This is decerebrate posturing; it results from a midbrain or pons lesion.
10. c Cerebral aneurysms generally rupture into the subarachnoid space of the basal cisterns.
11. c 4 to 14 days is the most common period for vasospasm.
12. a Cervical level injury results in impaired respiratory function.
13. d Voiding is the only choice that is affected by a sacral injury.
14. b AVM is a tangled collection of dilated vessels that allows blood to flow directly from artery to vein with no communicating capillaries.
15. d Increased oxygen demand, decreased chest wall movement, obstruction by the glottis, and increased bronchial secretions can all lead to respiratory distress in status epilepticus.

Matching—Cranial Nerves

1. d
2. c
3. g
4. a
5. l
6. h
7. b
8. i
9. e
10. j
11. f
12. k

Chapter 10 Crossword

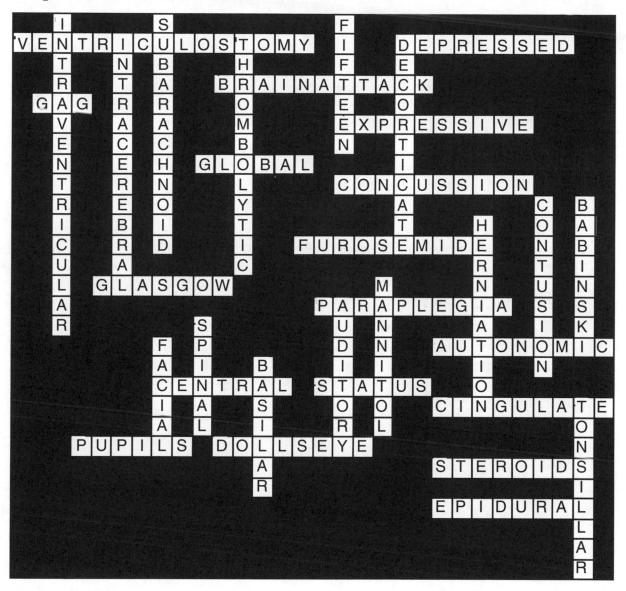

CHAPTER 11

True/False

1. T
2. F PaO_2 decreases, not $PaCO_2$.
3. T
4. F These are early indicators of hypoxemia associated with ARDS.
5. F Small tidal volumes (< 10 ml/kg) are recommended to prevent barotrauma.
6. T
7. F ARDS patients require 1.5 to 2 times the normal caloric intake.
8. T
9. T
10. F Aspiration of bacteria from the oropharynx and GI tract typically causes VAP.

Multiple Choice

1. c After long exposure to high CO_2 levels, the baroreceptors respond only to hypoxia as a stimulus for breathing.
2. a The purpose of pursed lip breathing is to exhale slowly, which allows air trapped in the alveoli to escape.
3. b Atelectasis means collapsed alveoli, which prevents normal bronchovesicular sounds.
4. d Neurologic signs and changes in LOC are the initial symptoms seen in impending ARF.
5. d Intrapulmonary shunting occurs when areas of the lung are inadequately ventilated but adequately perfused.
6. b CO_2 diffuses more readily than O_2, so hypoxemia results first.
7. b The lower and upper airways do not play a part in gas exchange; this is normally 25%–30% of the inspired volume.
8. b Hypocapnia results from tachypnea as the patient tries to increase his or her PaO_2.
9. b A COPD patient who chronically retains CO_2 may have baseline ABGs that show both PaO_2 and $PaCO_2$ in the 50–59 mm Hg range.
10. d Vichow's triad includes venous stasis, disease states that alter coagulability, and damage to vessel walls.

Symptom Identification

1. E
2. E, L
3. L
4. L
5. E
6. L
7. L
8. E
9. L
10. L
11. L
12. E, L
13. E
14. E
15. L
16. L
17. E, L
18. L
19. E
20. L

Chapter 11 Crossword

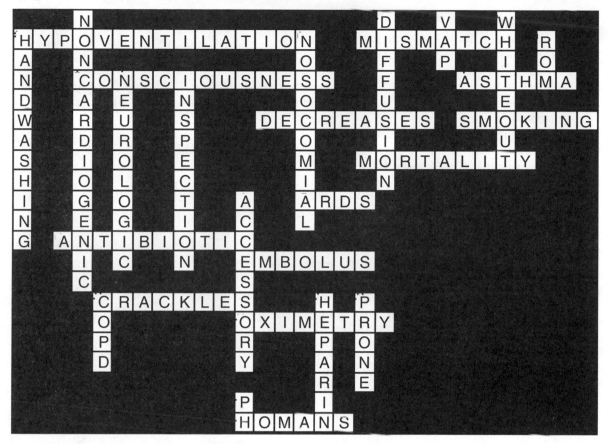

CHAPTER 12

True/False

1. F Hyperkalemia is the most life-threatening complication of ARF, because it can cause fatal dysrhythmias.
2. F A major goal of nutritional management in ARF is to reduce catabolism of protein, which results in increased urea, phosphate, and potassium.
3. T
4. F Nonoliguric patients may excrete this amount of urine in 24 hours, but the urine is deficient in the solutes and waste products that compose normal urine.
5. F Hemodialysis is the most frequently used renal replacement therapy. CCRT is often used for patients in the ICU whose cardiovascular status is too unstable for the rapid fluid removal of dialysis.
6. T
7. F Peak and trough levels are done in ARF because of the need to adjust medication dosages in order to avoid accumulation side effects which occur as a result of dysfunction of the kidney.
8. T
9. F Renal anemia is caused by decreased production of erythropoietin. Treatment with erythropoietin is effective but may lead to a functional iron deficiency because of increased demand for iron to support erythropoiesis.
10. F If needed, intermittent catheterization, not indwelling, is recommended using strict aseptic technique.

Multiple Choice

1. c. Fluid restriction is often matched to urine output volume in 24 hours plus insensible losses (about 600–1000 ml/day).
2. b. Normal creatinine clearance is 125 ml/min, so a value of 5 ml/min is consistent with renal dysfunction.
3. b. Excessive urea and increased ammonia produced by bacterial breakdown of urea result in GI irritation, stomatitis, and a metallic taste in the mouth, all of which contribute to altered nutrition.
4. b. An elevated BUN has an antipyretic effect.
5. c. During the initiation phase, from the primary event to the beginning of the change in urine output, ATN is potentially reversible.
6. c. Postrenal obstruction may require a ureteral stent if the obstruction is due to calculi or carcinoma.
7. c. Sodium is measured in relation to water, so hyponatremia is often the result of water excess, which is treated with fluid restriction.
8. b. Metabolic acidosis in ARF results from the inability of the kidney to excrete hydrogen ions and synthesize bicarbonate. Rate and depth of respirations increase in an effort to compensate for the metabolic acidosis.
9. b. Complications from dialysis include all except hypertension. Hypotension occurs in 10%–50% of patients and is usually caused by preexisting hypovolemia, excessive fluid removal, or too rapid removal of fluid.

Matching—Key Terms

1. f
2. j
3. h
4. b
5. d
6. i
7. a
8. e
9. c
10. g

Chapter 12 Crossword

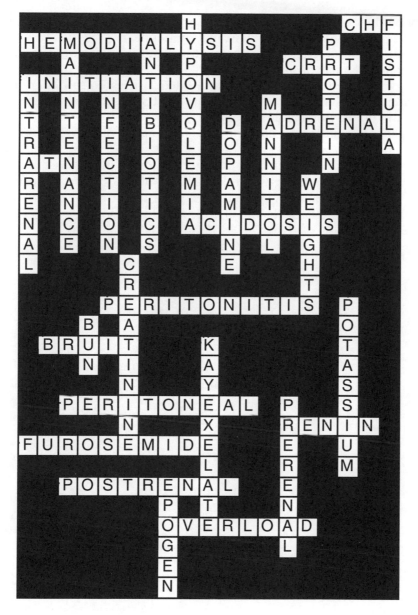

CHAPTER 13

Multiple Choice

1. d IgM is the major early antibody, followed by IgG. Others peak and recede at different intervals during the immune response.
2. b Fatigue, dyspnea, and tachycardia all result from insufficient oxygenation of tissues in anemia.
3. c Tissue hypoxia is the stimulator for erythropoiesis.
4. d Vitamin B_{12} deficiency causes demyelination of peripheral nerves to the spinal cord.
5. a Spontaneous bleeding may occur at 20,000–30,000/mm^3. Levels above 50,000 rarely cause significant complications.

6. a   Humoral immunity is mediated by B lymphocytes; cellular immunity is mediated mainly by T lymphocytes.
7. a   Fever may be the only sign of infection present. In neutropenia the WBCs are decreased, and without phagocytosis, typical signs may not appear.
8. d   DIC often manifests as acral cyanosis; occult blood in stools, emesis, or urine; hypotension, hypoxemia, and acidosis.
9. d   All others are treatments for primary immunodeficiencies. In secondary immunodeficiency, treatment includes administering antiinfectives, correcting malnutrition, and alleviating the underlying condition.
10. b   Fibrinolysis means splitting up of fibrin. It is the natural dissolution of fibrin into fibrin degradation products.
11. d   Education regarding disease transmission and the course of the disease decreases isolation and fears and allows for better understanding of treatments and other concerns.
12. c   Single-donor platelet products expose the recipient to antigens from only one person, thus reducing chances for febrile and allergic reactions.

Matching—Key Terms

1. f
2. m
3. r
4. e
5. b
6. g
7. q
8. a
9. k
10. p
11. l
12. h
13. c
14. j
15. d
16. o
17. n
18. i

Matching—Blood Products

1. c
2. f
3. d
4. a
5. h
6. g
7. b
8. e

Chapter 13 Crossword

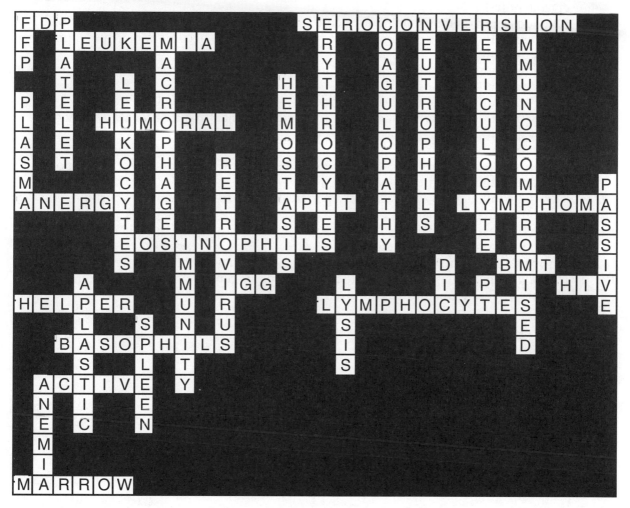

CHAPTER 14

True/False

1. T
2. F   Chyme is a semifluid mixture of food and gastric secretions.
3. F   Pepsin is active only in a highly acidic environment, with pH less than 5.
4. F   Vitamin B_{12} is absorbed with intrinsic factor, but in the terminal ileus.
5. T
6. T
7. T
8. F   A Mallory-Weiss tear is an arterial bleed from a longitudinal tear in the gastroesophageal mucosa.
9. T
10. T

Multiple Choice

1. b   Brunner's glands secrete mucus, which protects the duodenal wall from digestion by gastric juice.

2. d Needed glucose is formed by splitting glycogen stored in the liver; this is called glycogenolysis.
3. d All endoscopic therapies are performed to tamponade the vessel and stop active bleeding. Delayed surgery is performed in the case of a patient needing more than 8 units of blood in a 24-hour period.
4. a The most common complications leading to death in the first two weeks are pulmonary and renal complications.
5. c Lipase and amylase are released as pancreatic cells and ducts are destroyed.
6. d A low-protein, high-carbohydrate diet is ordered in small frequent meals to provide energy and to decrease nausea. Fats are typically avoided.
7. d All are important in preventing transmission of hepatitis.
8. d Kupffer's cells are phagocytic and in hepatic failure their function is lost, predisposing the patient to severe infections.
9. b Metabolic imbalances associated with pancreatitis are hypocalcemia, hyperlipidemia, hyperglycemia, and metabolic acidosis.
10. c Up to 10 liters of fluid enters the GI tract daily, including saliva, gastric and pancreatic juices, bile, and intestinal secretions.
11. a Vasopressin is a synthetic antidiuretic hormone that has direct vasoconstrictive effects.
12. d *Helicobacter pylori* has been associated with the pathogenesis of various gastroduodenal diseases, including peptic ulcer formation.

Matching—Key Terms

1. g
2. b
3. j
4. h
5. a
6. c
7. f
8. e
9. i
10. d

Chapter 14 Crossword

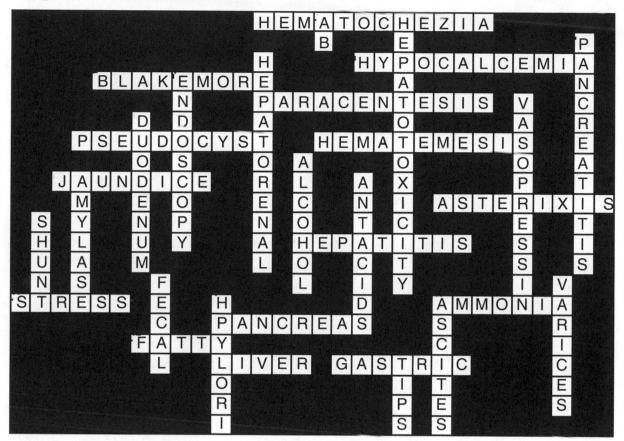

CHAPTER 15

Multiple Choice

1. b The osmotic diuresis that accompanies DKA (polyuria) leads to dehydration and electrolyte imbalances, causing polydipsia and abdominal pain. Acetone results from lipolysis and ketone formation, causing the "fruity" breath.
2. b Bicarbonate is decreased in DKA because of osmotic diuresis. Carbonic acid accumulates and the respiratory system attempts to compensate by blowing off CO_2.
3. b In HHNC there is no ketosis (or mild ketosis); osmolality and glucose are higher.
4. a Cortisol is released in response to ACTH release from the anterior pituitary as part of a negative feedback system.
5. d Choices a, b, and c are all primary causes of hypothyroidism.
6. c Somnolence, mucinous edema, weight gain and ascites occur with long-term hypothyroidism.
7. c Choices b and d are not electrolytes. Hyponatremia occurs with hypothyroidism as a result of water retention.
8. c Deficiency of aldosterone in primary adrenal crisis results in decreased sodium and water retention.
9. d Secondary DI is caused by excessive water intake, as in abnormal regulation of thirst or in mental illness.
10. c The hallmark of SIADH is hyponatremia and hypoosmolality in the presence of concentrated urine. Water retention is increased in SIADH.

Matching—Symptom : Hormone Level

1. f
2. b
3. h
4. c
5. a
6. e
7. g
8. d

Matching—DKA or HHNC

1. c
2. a
3. b
4. c
5. a
6. b
7. a
8. a
9. a
10. c
11. a
12. b
13. b
14. a
15. b

Chapter 15 Crossword

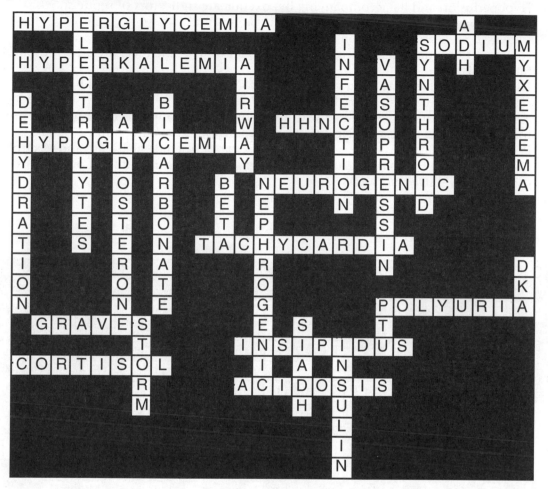

CHAPTER 16

True/False

1. F Traumatic injury is the leading cause of death in persons 1 to 44 years old.
2. F This is part of the primary survey, to provide a baseline for analysis of trends.
3. T
4. F Serum lactate levels increase in anaerobic metabolism, resulting in metabolic acidosis.
5. T
6. F Hypothermia, in combination with acidosis and coagulopathy, is associated with increased mortality.
7. F Intervention for a tension pneumothorax is never delayed for x-ray confirmation.
8. T
9. F Loss of sympathetic output following a spinal cord injury will cause hypotension and bradycardia.
10. T

Multiple Choice

1. c A level 1 trauma center provides the most sophisticated care; other facilities transfer to it.

2. c Stab wounds result in a direct path of injury.
3. c Hypoperfusion and its accompanying hypoxemia are indicators of septic shock.
4. c Blood products are not administered in the prehospital transport.
5. d Increased myocardial irritation is common among the elderly population.
6. c New-onset dyspnea, tachypnea, hypotension, and low-grade fever are all symptoms of a fat embolism.
7. a DPL can detect bleeding from within the abdomen, but it cannot reliably identify retroperitoneal bleeding from the kidneys or pancreas.
8. d Tension pneumothorax is treated with insertion of a 14-gauge needle into the second intercostal space, midclavicular line. Trapped air escapes, making a hissing sound.
9. c Potential complications of massive fluid resuscitation include acid-base and electrolyte imbalance, hypothermia, coagulopathies, organ dysfunction, and fluid overload syndromes (SIRS, MOF, and ARDS).
10. d Sepsis is an indirect cause of ARDS in trauma patients.

Chapter 16 Crossword

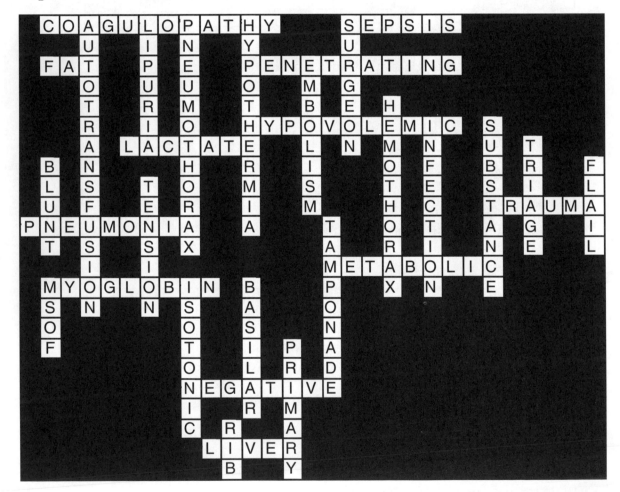

CHAPTER 17

Multiple Choice

1. a   Even if only 5% of TBSA has full-thickness burns, the patient should be transferred to a burn center.
2. d   The resuscitative phase lasts for about 48 hours and is the most crucial for the patient. The main goal is to prevent shock as fluid shifts occur.
3. c   Severe tissue damage causes release of chromagen. When chromagen is concentrated in small volumes of urine, renal failure can result.
4. c   A child's head is larger in proportion to lower extremity size than an adult's.
5. b   Coagulation is the site of irreversible skin death; hyperemia is the site of minimal cell involvement; stasis is potentially salvageable from cell death.
6. b   Vasoconstriction and further heat loss are not desirable; large amounts of body heat are already lost.
7. d   Clothing should be removed in a chemical burn injury because the chemical will continue to damage the skin (and respiratory tract) if left intact. Clothing is left on in thermal injuries.
8. b   Burns result in a massive shift of fluid into the interstitial spaces, causing hypovolemic shock. Pain would cause an increase in BP; psychogenic shock would come later; and internal hemorrhage is not caused by burns.
9. c   Preset formulas guide fluid resuscitation. Half of the total volume is given in the first 8 hours, one-quarter in the second 8 hours, and one-quarter in the third 8 hours.
10. b   Flexion problems, even contractures, occur with burn wound healing unless aggressive physical therapy is done to prevent them.
11. c   Silver nitrate is effective against a wide spectrum of wound pathogens and fungal infections.

Matching—Burn Wound Care

1. d
2. f
3. g
4. b
5. a
6. e
7. c
8. h

Chapter 17 Crossword

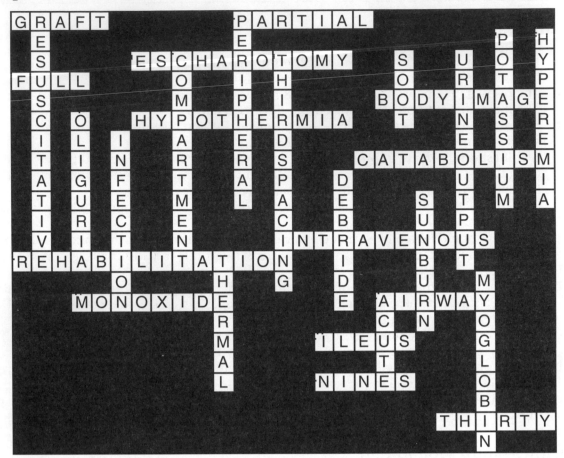